Shared Care
for ENT

Shared Care for ENT

Chris Milford FRCS
Consultant Otolaryngologist, Department of Otolaryngology,
The Radcliffe Infirmary
Woodstock Road, Oxford, UK

Aled Rowlands MB ChB
Family Practitioner, Montgomery House Surgery,
Bicester, UK

I S I S
MEDICAL
M E D I A

© 1999 by Isis Medical Media Ltd.
59 St. Aldates
Oxford OX1 1ST, UK

1st published 1999

British Library Cataloguing in Publication Data.
A catalogue record for this title is available from
the British Library

ISBN 1 899066 69 1

**Always refer to the manufacturer's Prescribing
Information before prescribing drugs cited in this book.**

Isis Medical Media staff
Commissioning Editor: John Harrison
Senior Editorial Controller: Catherine Rickards
Production Manager: Julia Savory

Page layout, design and reproduction by
Atlas Mediacom Pte Ltd, Singapore

Printed and bound by
Craft Print Pte Ltd, Singapore

Distributed in the USA by
Books International Inc., P. O. Box 605,
Herndon, VA 20172, USA

Distributed in the rest of the world by
Plymbridge Distributors Ltd., Estover Road,
Plymouth, PL6 7PY, UK

Contents

	Foreword	vi
	Preface	viii
	Introduction	x
Chapter 1	ENT examination	1
Chapter 2	The ear	21
Chapter 3	The nose	85
Chapter 4	The mouth and throat	109
Chapter 5	Injuries, emergencies and mandatory referrals	149
Chapter 6	Practical procedures in family practice	167
Chapter 7	Shared care in practice: case studies	173
	Index	189

Foreword

Excluding patients with upper respiratory tract infections, a typical general practitioner in the United Kingdom will see twelve patients in a week with an ENT problem. Despite this, very few aspiring general practitioners will undertake any formal training in ENT within a hospital setting.

Because the range of problems seen in a typical ENT outpatient clinic is very different from the ENT problems seen in primary care, it might be reasonable to argue that formal hospital-based ENT training may not be the best preparation for primary care; unfortunately, this is an argument that could be applied to many hospital posts that have traditionally enjoyed a place in the vocational training of general practitioners.

A common answer to this dilemma is to fill this training gap with a book. And here is one such book. So why should anyone consider this book in preference to any other? I think that the reasons are two-fold.

Firstly, the authors, Chris Milford (a Consultant ENT Surgeon) and Aled Rowlands (a General Practitioner with particular expertise in ENT problems) started off with the premise that sharing the care of patients with ENT problems between the primary and secondary care settings offers major potential advantages to the patient. If you are to write a book using that premise, you need to clarify what should rightly be dealt with (and how) within primary care, what should rightly be dealt with in secondary care, and what requires joint work. The authors manage to do this. At a time when the place of the referral process seems to be becoming more murky, this book offers a clear approach to both the methods and the setting of the best management of ENT problems.

Secondly, the authors have deliberately written the book to help the reader solve problems. The chapters deal specifically with common, or worrying, presentations, and then work the reader through to a solution. There is now a body of evidence to demonstrate that a problem-solving approach is more likely to help doctors alter their behaviour. It is commendable, therefore, that this is the approach the authors have taken.

I believe that this book deserves consideration by most general practitioners, but I think that it deserves a particular place on the shelves of the libraries of practices in which doctors are trained. But, unlike many books that are placed in libraries, my suspicion is that this one will spend a considerably greater proportion of its life being used. It deserves to!

Neil Johnson
Director of Postgraduate General Practice Education
Oxford, June 1998

Preface

There are many ENT textbooks currently in print that are primarily intended for medical students, junior ENT doctors and nurses but which are also said to be 'useful' for family practitioners. Almost without exception they are not problem-orientated, but deal with the subject on the basis of individual diseases, simply listing the various pathologies and describing their presenting signs, symptoms and management. Unfortunately, this is not how patients present to their family practitioners. In addition, these textbooks have been written by ENT specialists alone, and hence are written entirely from a hospital perspective. The spectrum of disease seen by a hospital specialist is very different from that seen by a family practitioner. It would seem an impossible task for an ENT specialist alone to provide a sense of perspective on the range of ENT problems likely to be seen in family practice, or to provide a range of protocols for the management of these patients.

We feel that there is a place for a textbook aimed exclusively at the family practitioner, written by both a family practitioner and an ENT surgeon. We hope we have created a text that is problem-orientated and can easily be used as a reference for the diagnosis and management of common ENT problems presenting in family practice. In particular, we have provided guidelines as to when and whom the family practitioner may need to refer on for further assessment, and to which patients can be managed safely within the surgery.

We have approached each of the problems dealt with in this book from our own areas of expertise. The family practitioner author has dealt with the presentation and clinical diagnosis based on symptoms and signs. The specialist author has dealt with the hospital perspective in terms of investigation and management of the patient within the hospital setting, and has given details of surgical management and recent advances where it was considered appropriate. Together we have dealt with the crucial area of when and whom to refer, as this appears to be the crux of the shared care concept in the field of ENT.

In summary, we believe that encouraging more shared care in ENT will provide better management of ENT problems in both family practice and hospital clinics. We hope that this book will promote this idea by focusing on the following points:

1. The development of protocols for family practice management and hospital referral of ENT problems.
2. The development of protocols that provide guidelines for direct referral where appropriate to surgical waiting lists (e.g. for tonsillectomy) or to hearing aid and audiology departments.
3. The development of co-operative strategies for postoperative management of patients by family practitioners and specialists (e.g. more shared long-term follow-up).
4. Education and the updating of family practitioners' knowledge of ENT diseases and their treatment.

We hope that this will be a useful book to have in your surgery as a quick and concise reference to common ENT problems.

Chris Milford
Aled Rowlands

Introduction

The shared care concept

The concept of shared care in ENT is the joint management of ENT problems by the family practitioner and the ENT specialist, carried out in a way which will improve patient management, encourage more appropriate referral patterns and, as a consequence, provide better value for money from health care expenditure.

The aims of shared care in ENT are better clinical management of ENT disorders in family practice, better use of ENT specialist services and providing value for money through better use of resources.

Shared care is growing in popularity in these times of increasing budgetary restrictions in most health care systems, as it is likely to be more cost-effective. It may also permit those patients with the most need of specialist evaluation and intervention more rapid access to diagnosis and treatment by an ENT specialist. Over the last decade patients have faced increasing waiting times to be seen at ENT specialist clinics, and attempts to reduce the length of these have encouraged an increase in shared care strategies. This is clearly of benefit to patients as it should provide more rapid access to diagnosis and treatment by ENT specialists when needed. It is also more professionally satisfying for the family practitioner.

ENT problems have always been recognized as playing a major part in family practice, although it is difficult to place an exact figure on this. ENT disorders represent 10–20% of all family practitioner consultations, and studies have shown that referrals to ENT departments represent approximately 11% of all referrals. Despite this, the amount of time devoted to ENT in undergraduate education is negligible and, although many ENT departments now run family practitioner study days, postgraduate education in ENT for many doctors has involved nothing more than learning on the job.

Our aim in this book is to discuss ENT disorders as they initially present to family practitioners in the surgery, and so we have adopted a problem-solving approach. For each presenting problem the family practitioner author discusses the initial management, while the specialist author describes what the hospital has to offer. In doing this, protocols for the management of each group of problems are described. One of the primary goals of shared care in ENT is, therefore, to attempt to define more clearly which patients should be managed in family practice and which should be referred to the ENT specialist. As the management of ENT diseases has changed over the last decade, so have the respective roles of family practitioners and specialists.

Our involvement with shared care in ENT was born out of necessity in 1990 when we assumed responsibility for the one ENT clinic held each week at the hospital in Banbury. This hospital serves a population of 130,000, and we were receiving approximately 1200 new referrals each year. This outpatient workload was far greater than could be dealt with in the time available, so we examined ways of reducing it by transferring work back to the family practitioners, i.e. by encouraging and fostering the shared care concept. Several examples of shared care were developed in discussions with the local family practitioners, including the following:

1. The follow-up of children who had undergone grommet insertion was undertaken by their own family practitioners rather than by bringing them back to the ENT department. In Oxfordshire now most children who have undergone grommet insertion are followed up by their own family practitioners using agreed protocols which indicate when patients should be referred back to the ENT department. This enables children and parents to see family doctors who know them well and who see them locally, and allows outpatient time in the ENT department for other patients to be seen.

2. Direct access to the surgical waiting list for family practitioners for straightforward cases of patients requiring tonsillectomy. As a history of recurrent acute tonsillitis is the major factor in determining whether a patient should undergo surgery, it seems appropriate for the family practitioner (who is in the best position to validate that history) to be able to list a patient for surgery if it

is felt to be appropriate. Any complicated or equivocal cases can still be referred for an initial outpatient consultation.

3. Direct referral by family practitioners of older patients for hearing aids to the hearing aid department. Many studies have shown that in the elderly population the ENT specialist does little for a patient referred for consideration of a hearing aid, so direct access for family practitioners to the hearing aid department seems a sensible use of resources. The ENT specialist thus only becomes involved with younger patients with a hearing loss or with atypical cases.

The trends towards the earlier discharge of inpatients postoperatively and towards more day surgery will also encourage and/or necessitate more shared care in ENT. All instances of shared care require a period of discussion between the ENT specialist and family practitioners' representatives, the issue of guidelines or protocols, and educational back-up. The single most important aspect of this approach would seem to be an attempt to give family practitioners some guidelines as to whom and when to refer on to the ENT department when dealing with common ENT problems, i.e. to help to identify those patients who may safely be managed by family practitioners and those who should be referred for specialist evaluation.

The ultimate goal of shared care in ENT is to enhance patient care both by improving understanding of these diseases and by fostering closer links between family practitioners and ENT specialists. This may result in greater satisfaction as far as family practitioners are concerned, in reduced time and money spent on inappropriate referrals, and in ENT specialists having more time to dedicate to those patients in whom specific intervention can make an impact on their quality of life. Most important of all, patients themselves will benefit from an increasingly more efficient and appropriate referral and treatment pattern.

Chris Milford
Aled Rowlands

Chapter 1

ENT
examination

Examination of the ear

Pinna and surrounding skin

The pinna and surrounding skin can be readily examined without the
use of instruments. It is useful to exclude tenderness of the pinna
(common in otitis externa) by moving the pinna and pressing on the
tragus.

Operation scars are often difficult to detect because of their
positioning in skin creases. Postaural and endaural (situated in the
groove between tragus and helix) scars (Figure 1.1) usually indicate
previous middle ear and/or mastoid surgery.

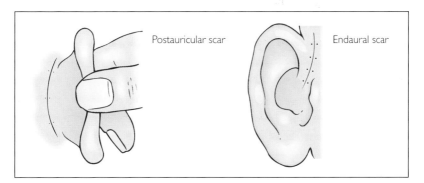

Figure 1.1 *Position of scars related to ear surgery.*

External ear canal

In many patients it is possible to see right down the ear canal as far as the eardrum if the external ear canal is straightened by holding the tragus forward with the thumb and pulling the pinna outwards. An angled light or headlight may be used for illumination.

Use of the auriscope: satisfactory examination requires adequate lighting and this is best provided by a fibreoptic auriscope (Figure 1.2) powered by rechargeable batteries. Once these batteries start to fade they lose power quickly compared to the gradual loss of power seen with conventional batteries, and their use avoids perhaps weeks of examining ears with an inadequate light source.

It is best to hold the auriscope like a pen. The little finger should be extended and used to anchor the examining hand on the face. The right hand should hold the auriscope to the right ear and the left hand to the left ear. It is then much easier to direct the auriscope into the canal, and the free hand can be used to pull the pinna outwards, so straightening the canal. The largest speculum that is comfortable should be used, as this provides the greatest illumination.

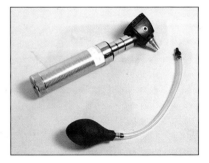

Figure 1.2 *A fibreoptic auriscope with pneumatic attachment.*

Tympanic membrane

Once the ear canal has been fully assessed to check for occlusive wax, signs of infection or polyps, it is essential to examine the entire tympanic membrane (Figure 1.3). The handle of the malleus should be identified first and followed up

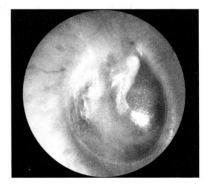

Figure 1.3 *The normal tympanic membrane.*

to its short, lateral process. The pars flaccida (attic area) is above this and the pars tensa below. Each should be examined in turn.

■ Does the attic area look normal, or is there evidence of disease such as retraction, erosion, crusting of old debris, or obvious cholesteatoma? Persisting wax in the attic area may be the only evidence of pathology.

■ Does the pars tensa look normal and translucent with visible middle ear ossicles, or is it dull and featureless?

■ Is the eardrum mobile? This can be assessed using the pneumatic attachment to the auriscope, making sure that the auriscope speculum forms a tight seal in the ear canal. Alternatively, watch the eardrum whilst asking the patient to perform the Valsalva manoeuvre: outward movement of the eardrum should be visible as the manoeuvre is performed. If the eardrum is immobile then the Eustachian tubes are not functioning, there is a middle ear effusion or there is a small perforation which can not be seen.

Examination of hearing

There are four factors for the family practitioner to evaluate in an individual with a hearing loss.

Severity of the loss: this is assessed clinically by free field speech testing (conversational and whispered voice testing) and audiometrically by pure tone audiometry.

Type of loss, which may be:

■ conductive, resulting from impairment of the passage of sound anywhere from the pinna to the stapedial/oval window joint

■ sensorineural, resulting from lesions affecting the cochlea, the audiovestibular nerve or the higher auditory pathways

■ mixed, as often both types of hearing loss are present. For example, patients with otosclerosis may have a sensorineural component to their hearing loss from cochlear damage, as well as the expected conductive loss from fixation of the stapes.

Pathology causing the loss: clinical examination may help to determine the cause of conductive hearing loss. Aetiological factors responsible for a sensorineural hearing loss may be identified from the history (prematurity, birth trauma, family history, exposure to noise trauma, head injury and ototoxics). In many cases of sensorineural loss no specific cause is identifiable.

Handicap caused by the loss: the family practitioner is in an ideal position to discuss with the patient the disabilities that the hearing loss has created.

Clinical tests of hearing in family practice and community health: young children

The importance of early diagnosis of hearing loss in children is well accepted, as are the potential benefits of early intervention in minimising the resulting disability, which can affect not only language but also social and emotional development. The aims of the community paediatric and child health services are to identify all children with significant hearing loss. One specific national objective is to identify 80% of all children with severe sensorineural hearing loss by the age of 12 months.

From birth to about 6 months the only reliable method of testing is in the ENT department by evoked response audiometry — an evoked potential in the eighth nerve, brain stem or auditory cortex may be recorded using skin electrodes following acoustic stimulation.

Distraction test: in the UK it is routine for children to have a hearing assessment as part of the developmental checks carried out by health visitors. The first test is the distraction test, performed at 6–7 months. At this age the child can sit with some support and with sufficient neck control to turn to sound.

The health visitor stands behind the child and presents the following three sounds to each ear in turn:

- high frequency – Manchester rattle (6000–10,000 Hz)
- middle frequency – 'sss' sound (4000 Hz)
- low frequency – hummed voice (250–1000 Hz).

These sounds are presented at 35 dB loudness as checked with a sound meter. About 25% of children fail this first test, which is then repeated one month later. If this second test is also failed then the child is either referred for the family practitioner to check the external and middle ears, or is referred directly to the paediatric audiology department by the health visitor.

Children who are not babbling loudly by the age of 9 months or responding to familiar words (e.g. their own names) by the age of 12 months should be considered to have a possible hearing loss.

Co-operative/performance tests can be used by health visitors and community audiologists to assess any child aged between 18 months and 4 years whose hearing is suspect. The child is asked to carry out simple tasks when he or she hears a noise. For example, in the *toy test* the child is presented in turn with 10 phonetically balanced names of toys to pick up. The voice is presented at 35 dB loudness.

Hearing is again tested by community audiologists just after the child starts school. This is done because it may be difficult to exclude unilateral, high frequency, sensorineural hearing loss with the earlier tests, and also to exclude deafness acquired in the intervening years and progressive deafness of congenital origin.

Clinical tests of hearing in family practice and community health: older children and adults

Free field speech testing, which can be carried out with patients over 5 years old, provides a guide to the level of hearing impairment. It involves establishing the threshold of hearing by asking the patient to repeat words that are spoken to him or her. It must be performed without giving the patient any visual clues, and it is necessary to mask the non-test ear (i.e. prevent the non-test ear from hearing). This may be done simply by massaging the tragus of the non-test ear while simultaneously asking the patient to repeat words spoken to the ear under test.

The loudness of the voice may be varied in two ways. In the first, the distance from the test ear may be altered. A patient with normal hearing in a quiet room should easily hear test words at arm's length (2 feet or 60 cm) — about as far as one can stretch whilst masking the non-test ear. If a whispered voice at arm's length cannot be heard, then the patient has a hearing impairment. Secondly, the level of the voice can be raised from a whisper to a normal conversational level and then to a loud voice. To a rough approximation, a whisper is about 30 dB and a conversational voice is about 60 dB.

Tuning fork tests (Figure 1.4) are generally underused in family practice. However, by using them a family practitioner should, in most cases, be able to decide whether the patient has a conductive or a sensorineural hearing loss, and should also be able to exclude cases of unilateral sensorineural hearing loss that would require further investigation to exclude serious pathology such as an acoustic neuroma.

The tests should be carried out using a 512 Hz fork — a 256 Hz tuning fork assesses vibration sense and therefore has no place in the testing of hearing.

The **Rinne test** assesses air conduction (AC) when the fork is held 5 cm from the ear (with the prongs in line with the ear canal), or bone conduction (BC) when the heel of the fork is placed on the mastoid bone behind the ear. It may help to determine whether a hearing impairment has a conductive component. The patient should be asked if the sound is louder when the fork is placed *beside* the ear or on the mastoid process *behind* the ear. In the patient with normal hearing or with a sensorineural hearing loss, the Rinne is *positive* (i.e. loudest beside the ear). The Rinne is *negative* when the fork sounds loudest behind the ear. This is typical of a conductive hearing loss of

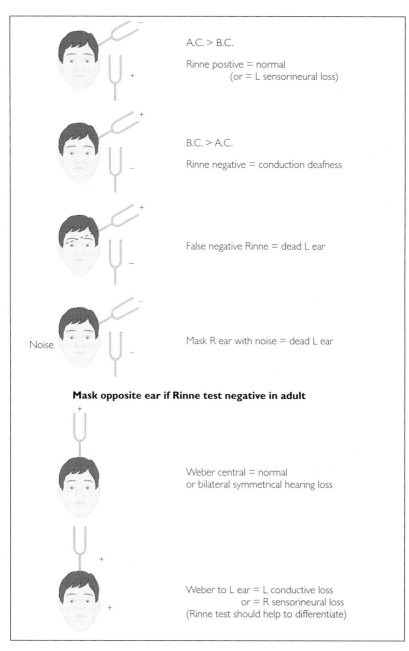

Figure 1.4 *Tuning fork tests of hearing — Rinne and Weber tests.*

greater than 20 dB.

A *false negative Rinne* may occur if the patient has no cochlear function ('dead' ear) on one side. In this situation, when the fork is placed beside the test ear (i.e. the ear with no function) it will not be heard. When it is placed on the mastoid behind the test ear the patient will hear it as the sound crosses over to be heard by the opposite normal cochlea. It will seem that the Rinne is negative suggesting a conductive loss. To avoid this mistake it is necessary to mask the non-test ear during testing (e.g. by massaging the tragus of the non-test ear) and then the fork will be unheard both beside *and* behind the ear.

In the *Weber test* the tuning fork is placed on the vertex and the patient is asked to indicate in which ear, if any, the noise sounds loudest. Normally the sound is perceived in the midline ('all over').

- If one ear has a sensorineural deficit, the sound lateralizes to the better hearing ear.
- If a conductive loss is present on one side then the sound goes to the side of the conductive loss, because surrounding noise will have less of a masking effect on the deaf ear than on the normally-hearing ear.

In mild conductive deafness the Rinne test may be positive but the more sensitive Weber test may still lateralize to the affected ear.

The nature of the hearing loss is best assessed on the basis of a combination of the results of the Rinne and Weber tests.

- If the Rinne is negative and the Weber lateralizes to that ear, then the loss is likely to be conductive.
- If the Rinne is positive and the Weber lateralizes to the opposite ear, then the loss is sensorineural.

Audiometry: many practices own an audiometer and train a practice nurse or a receptionist to carry out the test. This provides extremely useful additional information for the family practitioner in assessing the patient's hearing, and may indicate that referral for further more accurate audiological testing is necessary.

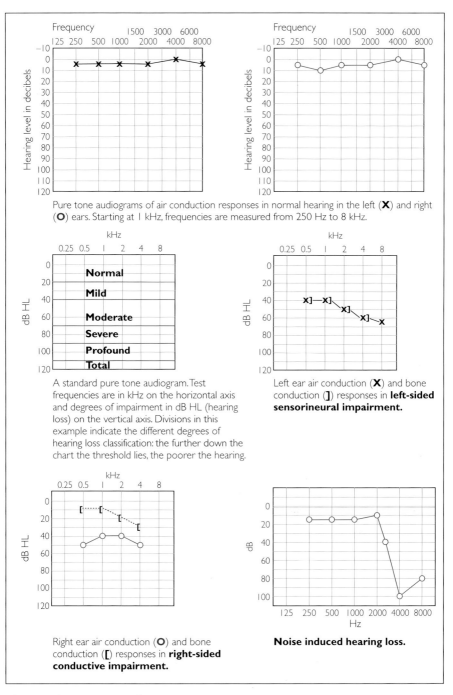

Pure tone audiograms of air conduction responses in normal hearing in the left (**X**) and right (**O**) ears. Starting at 1 kHz, frequencies are measured from 250 Hz to 8 kHz.

A standard pure tone audiogram. Test frequencies are in kHz on the horizontal axis and degrees of impairment in dB HL (hearing loss) on the vertical axis. Divisions in this example indicate the different degrees of hearing loss classification: the further down the chart the threshold lies, the poorer the hearing.

Left ear air conduction (**X**) and bone conduction (**]**) responses in **left-sided sensorineural impairment.**

Right ear air conduction (**O**) and bone conduction (**[**) responses in **right-sided conductive impairment.**

Noise induced hearing loss.

Figure 1.5 *Pure tone audiograms.*

Tests of hearing in the ENT department

Pure tone audiometry (Figure 1.5) is a subjective test and is unreliable in children under 4 years old. The aim of the test is to assess the ability of the patient to hear, i.e. to measure the threshold of hearing which is the least sound that the subject can just hear, and this should be explained to the patient.

By lowering and raising the sound level at which pure tones of different frequencies are presented, the thresholds of hearing (Table 1.1) can be assessed both by air conduction (through headphones) and bone conduction (using a special speaker applied to the mastoid bone).

- If the air and bone conduction thresholds are similar, the impairment is sensorineural.
- If the bone conduction thresholds are better than the air conduction thresholds there is a conductive defect.

Impedance audiometry or tympanometry (Figure 1.6) measures movement of the eardrum and ossicular chain and is, therefore, affected by the stiffness of the eardrum itself, the state of the middle ear and the stiffness of the ossicular chain. The ear canal is sealed off with a probe with three holes.

Table 1.1 Degree of hearing loss classification

- Normal   0–20 db
- Mild   20–40 db
- Moderate   40–70 db
- Severe   70–90 db
- Profound   90–110 db

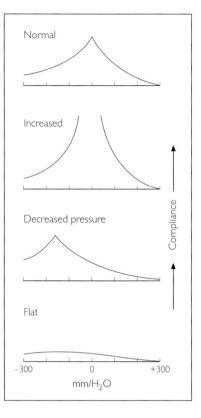

Figure 1.6 *Tympanometry: the four most common types of trace.*

- Through one hole a pure tone is introduced using a speaker.
- Through a second the pressure in the ear canal can be varied, so altering the tension of the eardrum.
- A microphone in the third picks up the reflected sound.

Most sound is absorbed when the external ear canal pressure is the same as that in the middle ear. By varying the pressure, graphs of compliance are obtained whose peak indicates the middle ear pressure.

Causes of a flat trace (i.e. a trace without a peak) include:

- fluid in the middle ear
- wax in the ear canal
- a perforation within the eardrum
- a patent grommet within the eardrum.

Key points

- 80% of all children with severe sensorineural hearing loss should be fitted with hearing aids by the age of 12 months.
- Patients who cannot hear whispered words at arm's length have a hearing impairment.
- A combination of the Rinne and Weber tests may determine whether the hearing loss is conductive or sensorineural in nature, but will not indicate the level of the hearing loss.
- The Rinne test is positive (AC>BC) in normal hearing or in sensorineural hearing loss.
- The Rinne test is negative (BC>AC) in conductive deafness.
- Beware of a false negative Rinne test, which may occur in a non-functioning ear unless the functioning ear is masked.
- Pure tone audiometry is the standard method of assessing hearing thresholds. It is a subjective test.
- Tympanometry is an objective test and may help diagnose negative middle ear pressure and otitis media with effusion (glue ear).

Examination of the throat and neck

Examination of the mouth

The mouth and oropharynx can readily be examined with a bright light and a tongue depressor (which can be used to retract lips, cheeks or tongue). All areas of the mouth should be examined and so patients should always be asked to remove their dentures. The examination should be performed systematically – starting with the lips, then moving onto the buccal surfaces, teeth, tongue (including its lateral borders), palate and tonsils.

Any visible lesion should be palpated for induration. Indeed, if the patient considers that there is something 'there', the suspicious area should be palpated even if no visible lesion is noted.

Examination of the larynx, pharynx and nasopharynx

Examination of the rest of the throat (nasopharynx, hypopharynx and larynx) requires the use of a mirror or endoscope. Even in experienced hands indirect laryngoscopy (Figure 1.7) provides adequate visualization of the larynx in only about 70% of cases. Flexible fibreoptic nasolaryngoscopy (Figure 1.8) permits a more thorough examination of all these areas, allowing a clear view of the nasopharynx, oropharynx, hypopharynx (that part of the pharynx behind the larynx) and larynx. The instrument is passed through the

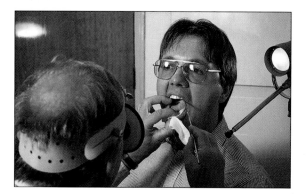

Figure 1.7
Mirror examination of the larynx (indirect laryngoscopy) in a cooperative patient.

nose under local anaesthetic (cocaine or lignocaine) and then via the nasopharynx, oropharynx and hypopharynx to allow visualization of the larynx. It permits good assessment of the larynx but does not always allow full assessment of the hypopharynx (sometimes a formal rigid endoscopy under general anaesthesia may be required).

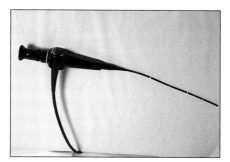

Figure 1.8 *A flexible fibreoptic nasolaryngoscope.*

Examination of the neck

The whole neck should be exposed and initially inspected from the front.

Palpation to detect any masses is peformed when standing behind the patient, flexing his or her chin downwards. The submandibular area, along the anterior border of the sternomastoid and the supraclavicular fossae should be palpated for any enlarged lymph nodes. A check should be made for movement of any masses on swallowing (any mass attatched to thyroid or larynx will move up on swallowing) and on moving the tongue (thyroglossal cysts move up on swallowing *and* on tongue protrusion).

If the mass is in the area of the submandibular gland then it should be palpated bimanually, using a gloved finger within the mouth with the other hand on the external surface, and assessing the mass between the two. The submandibular duct orifice (opening to the side of the frenulum beneath the tongue) should also be examined for evidence of pus or a stone.

If the mass is in the area of the parotid then the parotid duct orifice (opposite the upper second molar), the function of the facial nerve and the oropharynx (a lesion of the deep lobe of the parotid can cause distortion of the oropharynx) should all be assessed. It should be remembered that the tail of the parotid extends below the ear lobe, and *any mass around the ear lobe should be assumed to be within the parotid until proved otherwise.*

Normal anatomical structures may be mistaken for pathological masses. The following are often normally palpable:

- submandibular glands
- transverse process C2
- hyoid bone
- prominent carotid bulb.

Investigations in the ENT department: throat and neck

Radiology: radiological investigations may include the following:

- A lateral soft tissue neck X-ray may give information about soft tissue masses and radio-opaque foreign bodies.
- A barium swallow may be indicated in patients with swallowing problems.
- CT and MRI scans are most useful for documenting the position of tumours and abscesses, and for showing the involvement of related vital structures.

Other tests

- Throat swabs and a Paul-Bunnell or monospot blood test may be appropriate if a throat infection is suspected.
- Fine-needle aspiration cytology (FNAC) may be used in any neck lump in an attempt to provide a histological diagnosis. Its interpretation in the case of salivary gland pathology is more difficult.
- An upper aerodigestive tract rigid endoscopy under general anaesthesia is necessary where clinical suspicion of serious pathology exists.

Key points

- Never excise a small lesion around the ear lobe without considering whether it could be within the parotid (masses within the gland can feel extremely superficial) and considering whether it involves the facial nerve. ENT surgeons use a facial nerve monitor when operating in this area.
- Never examine the parotid without testing facial nerve function.
- Assessment of the submandibular gland involves bimanual palpation.

Examination of the nose

External nose

External examination of the nose will detect anatomical deformities of the bony and cartilaginous skeleton. An external deviation may be related to a previous fracture of the nasal bones, or to a deviation of the cartilaginous nasal septum. Occasionally, by elevating the tip of the nose with the thumb, the nasal septum can be seen to be dislocated into the nasal vestibule on one side, appearing as a vertical, linear protrusion in the nasal mucosa.

Air flow

Air flow and patency of the nasal airways can be assessed by holding a cold tongue depressor just beneath the nasal vestibule and observing the misting pattern, or by placing a thumb underneath each vestibule and judging the air flow through the other side whilst the patient breathes in and out gently (Figure 1.9).

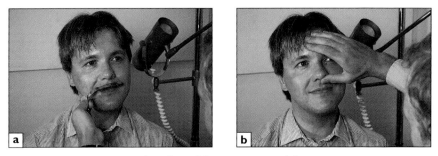

Figure 1.9 *Assessing nasal airflow. (a) Comparison of the misting pattern on a metal tongue depressor. (b) One thumb gently occludes the nostril and the patient is asked to breath gently in and out.*

Nasal cavity

The nasal vestibule can be inspected simply by elevating the tip of the nose with the thumb. In a child this may allow a complete examination without requiring a speculum.

Examination of the nasal cavities is greatly helped by the use of a Thudichum's nasal speculum (Figure 1.10). The speculum should be held firmly with the thumb and first finger of the left hand, with its spring controlled by the middle and ring fingers (Figure 1.11). The use of the speculum permits a systematic examination of the nasal cavities (Table 1.2).

An auriscope can also be used to examine the nose but the view obtained is not as good as when using a speculum. Patients should be told to hold their breath if the lens is in place.

A more detailed examination of the nasal cavity may be undertaken using a flexible or rigid (Hopkins' optical rod system) nasendoscope (Figure 1.12) and any patient referred to an ENT clinic with nasal symptoms is now likely to be examined in this way.

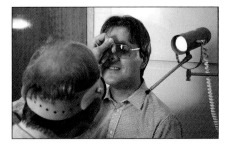

Figure 1.10
Anterior rhinoscopy. Gentle insertion of a Thudichum's speculum allows the anterior nose to be examined.

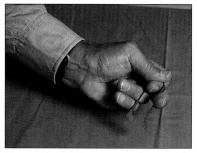

Figure 1.11 *Correct grip for use of Thudichum's nasal speculum.*

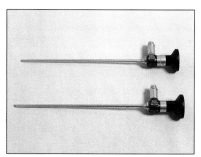

Figure 1.12 *Rigid nasal endoscopes (Hopkins' rod).*

Table 1.2 Systematic examination of the nasal cavities using Thudichum's speculum

- Does the nasal mucosa look normal (i.e. moist and pink)? Some secretions may normally be present.
- Assess the nasal septum. Is it deviated? Are there prominent vessels on the anterior nasal septum (Little's area, which is a common source of epistaxis in children)?
- Identify the inferior turbinate on the lateral wall of the nose. This is very prominent and often mistaken for a polyp, although they should be easily differentiated. When touched with a probe a turbinate is tender and immobile, whereas a polyp is not tender and is mobile.

	Pain	Mobile
Nasal polyps	-	+
Turbinates	+	-

- Look for mucopus in the middle meatus above the inferior turbinate, which may indicate infection in the anterior group of sinuses.
- Look for nasal polyps, which are the prolapsed oedematous lining of the ethmoid sinuses. They appear as pale grey/white bags which obstruct the nasal cavities to varying degrees. Tumours are generally pinker and more friable and are unilateral. A unilateral polyp is neoplastic until proved otherwise.

17

Postnasal space

The postnasal space is a difficult region to view with a headlight and mirror. However, flexible and rigid endoscopes are now used to view this area and to assess the posterior nasal septum, posterior choana, Eustachian tube orifices and nasopharynx.

In children with suspected adenoidal hypertrophy a lateral X-ray of the nasopharynx may be helpful.

In adults it is important that the postnasal space is examined in the following conditions:

- persisting unilateral glue ear
- persisting nasal obstruction where there is no identifiable cause
- recurrent epistaxes with no identifiable cause, especially if associated with other nasal symptoms
- patients with persisting enlargement of the cervical nodes.

Investigations in the
ENT department: nose

Radiology

- Plain X-rays: information obtained from plain views of the paranasal sinuses is often limited and this investigation should not routinely be requested by family practitioners.
- CT scans (Figure 1.13): any patient referred to an ENT department would have a CT scan of the paranasal sinuses carried out if radiology was indicated. CT provides information about the anatomy in any individual patient, and indicates the extent of the inflammatory disease within the sinuses, as well as documenting the spread of a soft tissue mass into adjacent structures (e.g. the orbit).
- MRI may be helpful in differentiating tumours from retained secretions and assessing intracranial/intra-orbital involvement.

Allergy tests

■ Skin tests may identify an atopic individual, although they are not particularly specific.
■ The radio-allergosorbent test (RAST) measures allergen-specific serum immunoglobulin E and is more specific. It is expensive, has little role in routine family practice assessment, and is not widely used in ENT departments.

Other tests

■ Various ciliary function tests are available to assess muco-ciliary function but none are widely used in clinical practice at the moment.
■ There are no consistently reliable tests to measure nasal airflow. Rhinomanometry and acoustic rhinometry are useful research tools.

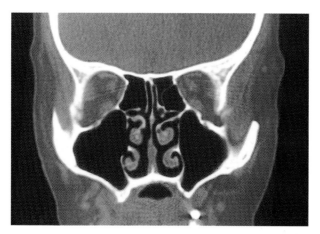

Figure 1.13 *A normal coronal CT scan of the sinuses.*

Key points

- Family practitioners should master the use of Thudichum's nasal speculum.
- Differentiate between polyps and turbinates by testing for tenderness and mobility.
- Mucopus in the middle meatus above the inferior turbinate may indicate infection in the anterior group of sinuses.
- A unilateral polyp is neoplastic until proven otherwise.
- The postnasal space must be examined in persisting unilateral glue ear in adults, and in persisting epistaxes and nasal obstruction where there is no identifiable cause.
- Plain X-rays of the paranasal sinuses should not be routinely requested.

Chapter 2

The ear

The external ear

The external or outer ear consists of the pinna and the external ear canal or meatus. It may be affected by congenital abnormalities and by any disease that affects exposed skin.

Congenital abnormalities of the pinna

Bat ears: abnormally protruding ears can make a child the object of derision from his or her peers. Pinnaplasty (pinning back the ears) is a simple procedure performed by many ENT and plastic surgeons, and should be considered for any child whose appearance causes concern.

Microtia: this describes any congenital deformity of the pinna. The severity of such deformities is very variable, ranging from a completely absent pinna through to an accessory auricle which is simply represented by a small skin tag anterior to the tragus. An accessory auricle will probably not require treatment. In the past, an absent pinna would have been treated with multiple plastic reconstructive procedures, but in recent years the use of osseointegrated implants has produced superior cosmetic results.

Preauricular sinuses are due to incomplete fusion of the primitive tubercles that form the pinna, and are usually sited just anterior to the tragus. They may be asymptomatic (in which case no treatment is required), but they can cause discharge and may become secondarily infected (Figure 2.1), in which case surgical treatment is indicated. A preauricular granuloma may be the only visible sign. Family practitioners should not be tempted to excise these under local anaesthetic as in rare cases they can extend deeply and be intimately related to branches of the facial nerve. An ENT specialist would use a facial nerve monitor when removing a skin lesion from the preauricular area, so it is unwise to consider this area as suitable for minor surgical procedures in family practice.

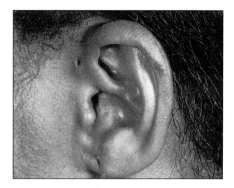

Figure 2.1 *A preauricular sinus. The small opening is clearly visible at the root of the helix.*

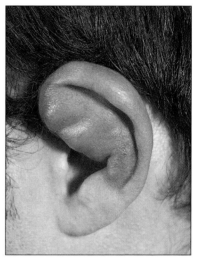

Figure 2.2 *Auricular haematoma.*

Other disorders of the pinna
Auricular haematoma (Figure 2.2) is a traumatic swelling caused by blood lifting the perichondrium away from the underlying cartilage. If this occurs on both sides, necrosis of the underlying cartilage results (especially if the haematoma becomes infected), giving rise to a cauliflower ear.

All patients require treatment unless the haematoma is small. The family practitioner should aspirate the haematoma, apply a pressure dressing and review the patient in 2 days. If aspiration is unsuccessful or if the haematoma recurs (as it often does), then referral is indicated as formal drainage is required.

Infection: perichondritis (Figure 2.3) usually follows trauma (including surgery) but can be secondary to any infection of the pinna. Cellulitis may complicate

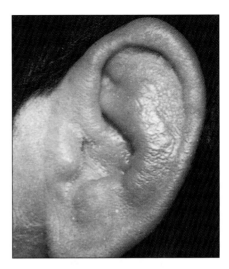

Figure 2.3 *Perichondritis.*

surgery, arise as a sensitivity to creams or ointments, or be secondary to an otitis externa. Perichondritis spares the lobule whereas cellulitis may involve it. The patient complains of a swollen, painful external ear which is painful to touch.

Referral is indicated if the patient does not respond quickly to a broad-spectrum oral antibiotic. Admission to hospital for parenteral antibiotics is likely in such cases, as inadequate treatment of perichondritis may result in the cosmetic deformity of a cauliflower ear.

Neoplasia: the development of basal cell and squamous cell carcinomas on the pinna is not unusual as it is one of the 'sun-exposed' areas. Any non-healing ulcer on the pinna should be viewed with suspicion and, if persistent, excised with an adequate margin for histology. It may be preferable to refer such patients.

The external ear canal

Congenital abnormalities: microtia may be associated with an absent ear canal and middle ear. Fortunately the inner ear is often normal, due to its different embryologic development. Assessment at an early stage is important, to allow hearing aids to be fitted if appropriate.

Trauma is often caused by the insertion of cotton buds or hairgrips, and results in laceration of the ear canal skin and bleeding. It may not be possible to see the eardrum to exclude injury, but even so it is usually reasonable to adopt a wait and see approach. Any blood clot should be left undisturbed and only treated actively if pain increases or discharge develops (antibiotic ear drops are more appropriate than oral antibiotics).

Normal findings on tuning fork testing can provide reassurance that ossicular injury is unlikely to have occurred. If audiology is available, a loss of greater than 60 dB might suggest such an injury and then referral may be wise. Although no immediate treatment would be planned by an otolaryngologist, if the hearing loss persisted there might be a case for exploring the ear at a later date to attempt to improve the hearing.

Foreign bodies inserted into the ear usually present in children and produce few symptoms except for blockage. Satisfactory removal requires skill, appropriate instruments and a good light source (although for non-vegetable foreign bodies syringing is sometimes appropriate), and if these are not available then referral is wise. It is likely that a child will only allow one attempt at removal and if this fails the foreign body will probably need to be removed under a general anaesthetic.

Wax: it is normal to have some wax in the ear canal — indeed it provides protection to the skin and possesses bactericidal activity. Ear canal epithelium migrates outwards, providing a natural cleaning mechanism for desquamated tissue and wax. Attempts by the patient to clean the ear invariably force the ear canal contents deeper into the meatus, resulting in impacted wax. The subsequent hearing loss is usually slight unless the wax completely occludes the ear canal.

Management involves syringing the ear canal, and once the wax has been removed the ear should be checked with an auriscope. It is important for anyone who may carry out the procedure (e.g. practice nurses) to be aware of the following contraindications to syringing:

- only-hearing ear
- history of perforated eardrum
- previous ear surgery
- recent trauma.

Infection: otitis externa is common.

Polyps arising from the middle ear may present in the auditory canal (Figure 2.4). They are usually secondary to chronic otitis media and may be attached to middle ear ossicles, so family practitioners should not be tempted to attempt

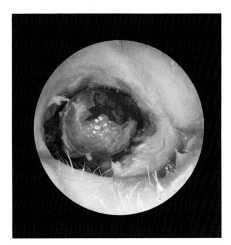

Figure 2.4 *An aural polyp within the ear canal.*

removal. These polyps are rarely malignant and are nearly always the result of prolonged suppuration. If the polyp is painful and bleeds, then malignancy is to be suspected, especially in the older patient.

Neoplasia: the common benign tumour arising from the ear canal is the osteoma. Arising from the deep bony ear canal, osteomas are hard and extremely sensitive if touched with a probe. They need no treatment unless they obstruct the canal and so give rise to symptoms.

Key points

- Auricular haematoma or suspected perichondritis require active treatment to avoid a long-term cosmetic deformity.
- Only attempt removal of a foreign body from a child's ear if you have the skills and instruments.
- Do not syringe out vegetable foreign bodies as they swell and impact in the ear canal.
- Wax is rarely a cause of a significant hearing loss unless it is obstructing the ear canal.
- Syringing is contraindicated following recent injury, where there is a history of perforated eardrum, or in an only-hearing ear.

Consider referring

- Auricular haematoma that recurs after aspiration.
- Perichondritis and cellulitis of the pinna which fail to respond quickly to oral antibiotics.
- Non-healing ulcers on the pinna.
- A child with a foreign body in the ear canal (unless confident of removal on the first attempt).
- Completely occluding impacted wax if syringing is contra-indicated.
- Preauricular skin lesions which require removal.
- Trauma to the ear where ossicular injury is suspected.

Otalgia

Pain in the ear is a very common presenting symptom and in most cases the diagnosis and management is straightforward. It may be related to a local problem associated with the ear itself, or it may be pain referred via one of several cranial nerves supplying the external and middle ears. A systematic approach is required: after taking a careful history, examination should initially be directed at finding an otological cause and then, in cases where there is no obvious ear disease, identifying a non-otological cause (Table 2.1).

Otological causes of otalgia

Otitis media: in children, otalgia is usually due to otitis media associated with an upper respiratory tract infection. In a study of pre-school children, the specificity and positive predictive value of earache for otitis media were 92% and 83%, respectively.

Chronic suppurative otitis media is usually painless but may be associated with pain if it leads to some of the complications associated with this disease.

Table 2.1 Otological and non-otological causes of otalgia

Otological causes
- Otitis media in children
- Complications of chronic suppurative otitis media (e.g. mastoiditis)
- Otitis externa
- Furunculosis
- Perichondritis
- Myringitis bullosa
- Acute otitic barotrauma
- Herpes zoster oticus (Ramsay Hunt syndrome)
- Neoplasia of the ear

Non-otological causes
- Tonsillitis
- Post-tonsillectomy
- Temporomandibular joint dysfunction
- Dental disease (e.g caries or abscess)
- Osteoarthrosis of the cervical spine
- Malignant disease of tonsil, pharynx or larynx

Otitis externa: symptoms are often bilateral and may vary from irritation to excruciating pain. Severe pain usually indicates cellulitis of the auditory meatus or pinna secondary to staphylococcal infection, and is an indication for systemic antibiotics in addition to topical antibiotic/steroid drops.

Furunculosis is infection of a hair follicle in the outer ear canal. Severe pain precedes rupture of the abscess. There may be significant swelling extending onto the tragus or pinna, and marked tenderness and pain on movement of any part of the cartilaginous meatal structure is typical. Any attempt to look into the ear with an auriscope causes severe pain, although it is often possible to insert a glycerine and icthamol gauze wick or an otowick soaked in antibiotic/steroid drops to ease the symptoms.

Perichondritis can follow severe otitis externa or be related to trauma. The infected cartilage produces a swollen, red, tender pinna. Systemic antibiotics are required to prevent damage to the cartilage which could result in a permanent residual deformity.

Myringitis bullosa is a localized form of otitis externa affecting the outer layer of the tympanic membrane. Haemorrhagic bullae form on the eardrum and deep meatus and present as severe otalgia. The condition is presumed to be related to a viral infection, but frequently proceeds to acute otitis media, and in rare cases to a viral labyrinthitis. Systemic antibiotic cover is generally advised.

Acute otitic barotrauma occurs during any rapid change in external pressure, e.g. when diving or descending in an aircraft. Failure of the Eustachian tube to open results in persistence of the low pressure in the middle ear, often with collapse of the eardrum and an accumulation of fluid. There may be bleeding into the ear and the patient complains of severe pain and has a conductive hearing loss. Any condition (e.g. a cold) that compromises

Eustachian tube function makes otitic barotrauma more likely, and so it is important to advise patients not to sleep when an aircraft is descending.

Herpes zoster oticus or Ramsay Hunt syndrome (Figure 2.5): the facial nerve ganglion may be affected by *H. zoster*, producing pain with associated vesicles in the ear canal and on the pinna. It may be accompanied by facial palsy. Treatment with aciclovir in the early stages may be beneficial.

Neoplasia of the ear: otalgia in these patients may be related to associated perichondritis or nerve involvement by tumour (Figure 2.6).

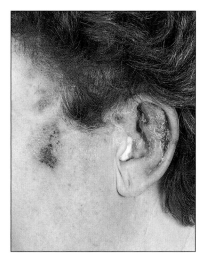 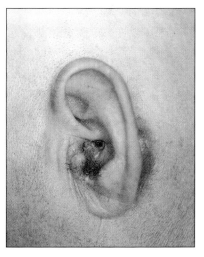

Figure 2.5 *Ramsay Hunt syndrome (*Herpes zoster *affecting the ear).*

Figure 2.6 *Carcinoma of the external ear canal.*

Non-otological causes of otalgia

The ear receives its sensory nerve supply from cranial nerves V, VII, IX and X, and the posterior roots of C2 and C3. If examination of the pinna, ear canal and eardrum is normal, otalgia is referred (Figure 2.7). In such cases its cause is frequently misdiagnosed and patients often receive unnecessary treatment with antibiotics and ear drops. Under these circumstances it is important to exclude a referred cause for the otalgia.

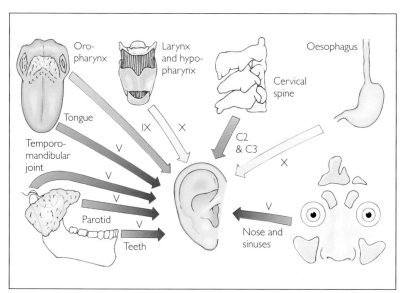

Figure 2.7 *Non-otologic causes of otalgia.*

Tonsillitis is the commonest cause for referred otalgia in children.

Post-tonsillectomy: otalgia is also very common after tonsillectomy, usually occurring 3–6 days after the operation. Antibiotics are not necessary.

Temporomandibular joint dysfunction and **dental disease** may cause otalgia in adults. The former causes tenderness over the temporomandibular joint and exacerbation of pain on opening the mouth or on chewing. Temporomandibular joint exercises may be helpful, but as there is often an associated malocclusion of the teeth, referral to an oral surgeon may be indicated if no improvement occurs.

Osteoarthrosis of the cervical spine can cause otalgia in the elderly.

Malignant disease: the most worrying cause of referred otalgia is that arising from a tumour of the tonsil, pharynx or larynx. It is usually accompanied by associated symptoms such as sore throat, hoarseness or dysphagia.

Key points
- Causes of otalgia may be otological or non-otological.
- Identification requires a systematic approach.
- Referred otalgia is frequently misdiagnosed.
- A tumour of the tonsil, pharynx or larynx is the most worrying possible cause of referred otalgia.

Consider referring
- Any patient with a local cause for otalgia who does not respond to standard therapy.
- Any patient with persistent unilateral otalgia where no local cause is identified, to establish that there is no serious pathology within the oropharynx, larynx and hypopharynx.

The discharging ear

Discharge from the ear (otorrhoea) is a common presenting problem in family practice, but diagnosing the cause can be difficult. It is likely to be due to disease of the ear canal or the middle ear (Table 2.2). As a first step in diagnosis and management, the discharging ear can be treated with ear drops (even when the tympanic membrane is perforated), with a reasonable chance of achieving a dry ear whatever the pathology. Even if a dry ear is not achieved using drops, the condition is often likely to improve sufficiently to enable examination of the ear canal and tympanic membrane, so assisting in diagnosis.

Table 2.2 Sources of discharge from the ear and possible diagnoses

Source of the discharge	Possible diagnosis
Ear canal	■ Otitis externa
Middle ear	■ Acute suppurative otitis media (ASOM) ■ Active chronic suppurative otitis media (CSOM) ■ Infected grommet ■ Infected mastoid cavity

Examination and diagnosis

Pain: severe earache is often the presenting symptom in acute suppurative otitis media (ASOM). Pain is caused by the build up of pus behind an intact tympanic membrane. Once the membrane ruptures and the pus starts to drain, the pain often improves or resolves.

Pain will also be a feature in severe otitis externa, and is often exacerbated by chewing (because movement of the temporomandibular joint distorts the ear canal) or by movement of the pinna or tragus. In this condition, pain will often be preceded by irritation.

If the ear is not painful, the most likely diagnosis is chronic suppurative otitis media (CSOM). In this condition, chronic perforation of the tympanic membrane allows any pus to drain into the ear canal, rather than build up behind an intact membrane.

Itching: basically dermatitis of the skin of the ear canal — usually indicates otitis externa.

Smell: a smelly discharge from the ear usually indicates CSOM with associated cholesteatoma, although it can sometimes be associated with otitis externa.

External auditory canal: the presence of swelling is diagnostic.
- Severe otitis externa often causes swelling of the external auditory canal, and sometimes this swelling extends to the pinna.
- Such swelling is unusual in CSOM unless the discharge has led to a secondary otitis externa.
- Swelling is also unusual in ASOM unless there is associated mastoiditis, when the posterior canal wall may swell and the roof sag, making examination difficult and painful.

Tympanic membrane: insertion of the auriscope may be painful and examination will reveal the discharge. If the discharge obscures the tympanic membrane, it should be cleaned away carefully with a cotton bud (or suction if available) to enable the membrane to be checked to see if it is intact. Commercial cotton buds are usually too large to be useful within the ear canal: home-made buds of cotton wool on a Jobson Horne probe may be more helpful. If suction is not available, careful syringing may clear the discharge. Syringing would not be used in an ENT department because of the availability of a microscope and suction, but it may be the only practical way of clearing the discharge. Syringing should only be used in family practice when it is clear that the tympanic membrane is intact. An alternative approach would be to prescribe ear drops and arrange a follow-up appointment in 1–2 weeks in the hope that the discharge settles enough to allow the membrane to be seen.

Once the tympanic membrane is visible, the handle of the malleus is usually the easiest structure to recognize. The membrane should then be checked. If it is unclear whether or not there is a perforation, the patient should be asked to perform a Valsalva manoeuvre — the membrane will move if it is intact. If there is a small perforation that cannot be seen, the membrane will not move and air bubbles may appear in the discharge (if enough is still present), or the patient may mention that they hear air 'escaping'.

Culture of the discharge is not usually helpful as the organisms grown are often contaminants. It is probably best reserved for resistant cases that do not respond to treatment.

Otitis externa

Most family practitioners will see one patient with otitis externa every fortnight. It has a large number of causes, including infection and allergy, and it may complicate skin conditions such as eczema and psoriasis in this area. Moist, humid environments predispose to ear canal infections and it is common for patients to have been abroad on a 'swimming' holiday before presenting with these conditions ('tropical ear', 'swimmer's ear'). In infective otitis externa, streptococci, staphylococci, pseudomonas and fungi (*Candida* and *Aspergillus*) are the usual infective agents.

Symptoms: the characteristic symptom of this condition is irritation. This can be intense and the patient may resort to scratching the ears with a variety of implements (such as cotton buds, matchsticks or hairgrips). Even if the condition has progressed to the point where the pain is severe, it will usually have been preceded by a period when irritation was the only symptom. When the ear is painful, the pain may be exacerbated by chewing, pressure on the tragus, or manipulation of the pinna. Hearing loss may be present and is usually mild and conductive in nature.

Examination: on examination, the ear canal is red and tender with an associated scanty discharge in the early stages (Figure 2.8). Later,

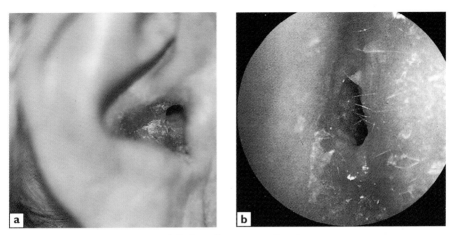

Figure 2.8 *Otitis externa. (a) Skin changes on the pinna. (b) View of the ear canal.*

pain and associated hearing loss may accompany a grossly oedematous ear canal (sometimes completely closing the ear canal) and this may obscure any view of the tympanic membrane. Debris and discharge may be present in the ear canal.

Treatment involves aural toilet — gentle dry mopping, gentle syringing or suction if available. Once clean, the ear should be treated with a combination of antibiotic and corticosteroid drops for 1–2 weeks and the patient should be advised to avoid:

- scratching the ears or using cotton buds
- getting water in the ears (e.g. by using cotton wool impregnated with petroleum jelly as ear plugs during hairwashing).

Most problems will resolve within 2 weeks using this treatment regimen.

If the ear canal is very oedematous, the drops may not penetrate the canal. In these circumstances, a dressing such as an otowick helps the drops to penetrate deep into the canal. An otowick is a firm, narrow sponge which is relatively easy to insert into the narrow

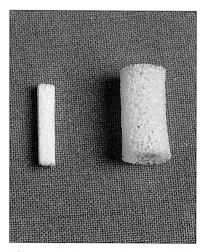

Figure 2.9 *An otowick, before (left) and after (right) the application of ear drops.*

ear canal and which expands when the drops are applied (Figure 2.9). The wick is kept moist with the drops and removed after several days. If pain or swelling prevents insertion of the wick, referral may be needed to clean the ear with suction using a microscope and to insert the wick. Otowicks can be useful for treating otitis externa in family practice, but are relatively expensive and cannot be prescribed on the NHS. This cost may be offset if referral is avoided.

If there is no infective element to the otitis externa and the irritation is slow to settle after treatment with the drops, then betamethasone lotion is often useful (particularly if the patient has a history of eczema).

Necrotizing (malignant) otitis externa: this is an aggressive inflammatory process which affects diabetic patients with small-vessel disease and immunocompromised patients. Although this condition starts as a localized otitis externa, it may progress to a spreading osteomyelitis of the skull base. A discharge is associated with pain which becomes progressively worse. On examination, there is usually granulation tissue along the floor of the ear canal as the bone of the canal becomes exposed. As the disease progresses, the osteomyelitic process leads to cranial neuropathies involving nerves VII, IX, X, XI and XII. Treatment involves prompt intravenous antibiotics with an agent such as ciprofloxacin, and the ear should be cleaned and dressed. Surgical debridement may be needed.

Any diabetic or immunocompromised patient with otitis externa that fails to respond rapidly to treatment probably warrants specialist referral.

Acute suppurative otitis media (ASOM)

ASOM is the commonest cause of a discharging ear seen in family practice. About 10% of children with ASOM will have an acute perforation of the tympanic membrane and discharge from the ear.

Symptoms: the overriding symptom is pain due to the build up of pus behind an intact tympanic membrane, and this is usually associated with deafness. Once the membrane ruptures and the ear starts to discharge, the pain resolves.

Examination: the appearance of the tympanic membrane is different at different stages of the condition.

- Initially, negative middle ear pressure causes acute pain, although the membrane usually appears normal (apart from slight retraction).

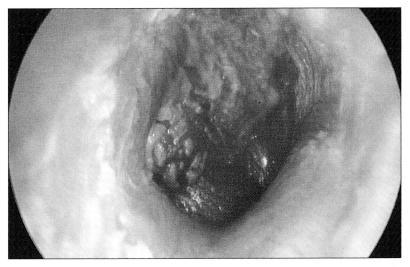

Figure 2.10 *Acute suppurative otitis media (ASOM): the whole membrane becomes red and thickened.*

- The earliest visible change is the appearance of dilated vessels in the membrane. It is important to remember, however, that the membrane of a crying child may show increased vascularity, and mild vascularity over the handle of the malleus is often normal.
- Later, the whole membrane becomes red and thickened and bulges — probably the most recognisable sign of ASOM (Figure 2.10).
- Finally, the membrane perforates and a purulent discharge is released.

Treatment: Most family practitioners in Britain treat acute otitis media with antibiotics. This is largely because bacterial pathogens (usually *Streptococcus pneumoniae, Haemophilus influenzae* or *Moraxella catarrhalis*) can be isolated from the middle ear in 60–70% of cases. However, the true value of antibiotics in this condition is uncertain. The number of well-conducted studies for this common condition is surprisingly small and most published papers have significant faults in methodology. Some studies have shown marginally better outcomes when measuring rates of resolution of some symptoms with antibiotic treatment.

No conclusion can be drawn from published work on the influence of antibiotics on the incidence of mastoiditis because:

- the numbers of patients in most studies are insufficient for analysing rare events (the incidence of mastoiditis is very low with or without antibiotics).
- in most studies treatment plans are promptly revised in children with persisting or recurrent symptoms and this precludes any conclusion as to whether the risk of suppurative complications is increased by witholding antibiotics.

In conclusion, therefore, the benefits of antibiotic treatment on short-term or long-term outcomes remain unproved, and it is appropriate that family practitioners discuss this with parents when considering whether or not to prescribe antibiotics for otitis media. If the family practitioner decides to prescribe an antibiotic then the choice lies between amoxycillin and second or third generation cephalosporins. Antibiotic concentrations in the middle ear decrease markedly during treatment and after the fifth day are usually of minimal therapeutic significance. This, taken together with the fact that 50% of patients fail to complete the full prescribed course, means that a 5-day course is usually adequate and there is some evidence that a 3-day course is just as effective.

Recurrent ASOM poses a difficult challenge to which there is no easy solution. The following activities may have a role in preventing ASOM recurring in susceptible patients:

- prophylactic antibiotic treatment to prevent the development of ASOM following viral upper respiratory tract infection
- regular, low-dose prophylactic antibiotic therapy over the winter months
- grommet insertion to reduce earache (although children may develop a discharge when they develop otitis media).

Grommet insertion should probably be reserved for severe cases or for patients who do not respond to or who are unable to take antibiotics.

Complications: over the last 30–40 years, the nature of ASOM has been altered by changes in the virulence of pathogens, improvement in the general health of the population, and the routine use of antibiotics. Complications are, therefore, seldom seen, but can include the following.

- Acute mastoiditis, which causes increasing pain and a decrease in the patient's general well-being. The area over the mastoid may be tender and the pinna may be displaced forwards and outwards, although these features can be difficult to distinguish from severe otitis externa and may be masked by previous antibiotic treatment.
- Labyrinthitis — occasionally infection can involve the inner ear, causing a sensorineural hearing loss and vertigo.
- Meningitis, cerebral/cerebellar abscess or lateral sinus thrombosis can be a result of intracranial spread of infection.
- Facial nerve palsy.

Follow up: it is difficult to justify reviewing all patients after an attack of otitis media. Most children have fluid persisting in the middle ear after each episode, and in 40% of cases this persists for up to 3 months. Significant effusions will present with deafness or recurrence of infection, and it may be preferable to alert the parents to this rather than reviewing every child. However, it is important to keep children with recurrent attacks under review, as they are likely to have persistent problems.

Active chronic suppurative otitis media (CSOM)

Active CSOM is associated with discharge and hearing loss, but seldom with pain. The classification of CSOM is difficult: it is traditionally categorized as either tubotympanic or attico-antral (Table 2.3).

Tubotympanic disease arises from bacterial infection and perforation of the central part of the tympanic membrane

Table 2.3 Comparison of tubotympanic and attico-antral CSOM

	Tubotympanic	Attico-antral
Symptom	Painless	Painless
	Profuse discharge	Scanty discharge
Position of perforation	Central	Attic/posterior marginal retraction or perforation
Cholesteatoma	Usually absent	Often present
Complications	Rare	Likely

following upper respiratory tract infections (Figure 2.11). Otoscopy reveals a perforation in the central area of the membrane (pars tensa). Medical treatment (aural toilet, a combination of antibiotic and corticosteroid drops, keeping the ear dry) often settles the discharge. If the perforation will not heal, surgical closure should be considered.

Attico-antral disease usually follows long-standing chronic, non-suppurative disease (often with chronic Eustachian tube dysfunction), resulting in retraction of the tympanic membrane in the attic or posterior segment (Figure 2.12). Otoscopy can be difficult, but will reveal a crust or perforation full of whitish debris (cholesteatoma) and a smelly discharge is usually present. A cholesteatoma is a slowly growing ball of skin-like epithelium which develops in the middle ear cleft and erodes the surrounding bone. It can damage the ossicles, facial nerve canal and extend into the bony labyrinth (inner ear), and intracranial suppuration can occur if the floor of the middle fossa is breached. Once the diagnosis of attico-antral disease is made, it is pointless continuing with medical treatment and surgery (some form of mastoid exploration) will be needed.

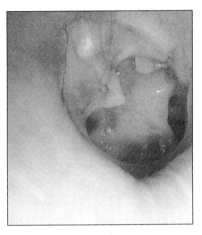

Figure 2.11 *Central perforation of the left tympanic membrane.*

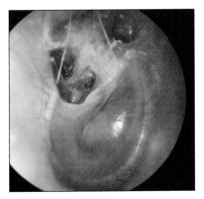

Figure 2.12 *Marginal perforation of the right tympanic membrane.*

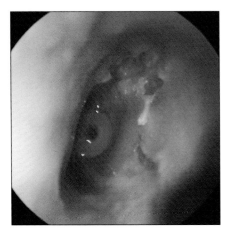

Figure 2.13 *An infected grommet.*

Other causes

Infected grommet: discharge is the commonest postoperative complication in children who have had a grommet inserted (Figure 2.13). In most cases, the discharge will settle with a course of ear drops. If the discharge does not settle, it is often worth trying a different type of drop, before referring for a specialist opinion. Occasionally, removal of the grommet will be the only way to achieve a dry ear.

Infected mastoid cavity: it is not uncommon for patients who have undergone mastoid surgery for cholesteatoma to have persistent or intermittent discharge from the cavity. Ear drops are likely to resolve the problem, but if persistent, the condition may need specialist referral for ear suction under microscopic guidance.

Assessment and management in the ENT department

In the UK, otitis externa is the commonest reason for referral. The hospital setting provides the advantage of easy access to a microscope and suction, and by removing the discharge under microscopic control, the ear canal and tympanic membrane can be inspected in all but the most severe cases. Even so, medical treatment with ear drops for 1–2 weeks followed by re-examination may be needed to allow full examination for a definitive diagnosis. The microscope allows the identification of perforations more easily than the auriscope, particularly if a discharge is present. It is almost essential to have access to a microscope and suction to treat a discharging mastoid cavity effectively.

If there is no perforation or evidence of cholesteatoma, then a diagnosis of otitis externa can be made by exclusion. In this situation, regular aural cleaning using the microscope together with the use of ear drops will resolve the problem in most cases, although some patients will develop recurrent problems in the future.

Key points

- The main causes of ear discharge are otitis externa, ASOM and CSOM.
- Profuse discharge suggests middle ear disease.
- In children who have a grommet inserted, infection of the grommet is the most likely cause of discharge.
- The history (does it hurt, itch or smell?) may be diagnostic.
- Examination involves cleaning the ear and assessing the integrity of the tympanic membrane. Syringing should only be used if the tympanic membrane is intact.
- Management basically involves aural toilet together with a combination of antibiotic and corticosteroid drops, whatever the underlying pathology. Ear drops can be used in patients with a perforated tympanic membrane for a limited period.
- Beware otitis externa in diabetic or immunocompromised patients.
- A smelly discharge suggests cholesteatoma.
- Earache or headache in patients with chronic ear disease suggests the possibility of intracranial complications.

Consider referring

Otitis externa
- Any patient whose condition has failed to respond to two courses of ear drops.
- Any patient in whom it is impossible to clear the ear canal because of large amounts of debris or marked oedema.
- Diabetic or immunocompromised patients with otitis externa.

ASOM

- Patients with persisting otorrhoea after treatment.
- Patients suffering from deterioration in general health despite treatment (to exclude complications).
- Patients suffering increasing pain despite usual treatment.

CSOM

- Patients with a smelly discharge (this suggests cholesteatoma).
- Patients with CSOM who develop increasing earache or headache (this suggests intracranial complications).
- Young patients with a persistent central perforation in whom surgical closure of the perforation is being considered (to reduce possible recurrent discharge from the ear).
- Patients suspected of having attico-antral disease.

Infected grommet or infected mastoid cavity

- Persistent discharge where the problem has not resolved with ear drops.

Hearing loss in children

Hearing loss or deafness is an impairment to communication at any age but is a major handicap to developing communication in children. Early detection and management are therefore essential if adequate speech and language are to develop. The incidence of severe sensorineural hearing loss in children is approximately 1 in 1000 and members of the primary health care team should suspect hearing loss in the at-risk groups (Table 2.4) and refer them for audiometric assessment.

The most common cause of hearing loss in childhood relates to middle ear disease, in particular to otitis media with effusion (OME), usually known as glue ear.

Table 2.4 Risk factors for hearing loss in children

- Birth factors: prematurity, low birthweight or neonatal jaundice
- Failed health visitor distraction test
- Parental suspicion of hearing loss
- Abnormal speech/language development
- Family history of deafness

Glue ear

At least one third of children of 1–8 years of age have recurrent episodes of OME. The peak incidence is at 2–4 years of age and the main symptom is hearing impairment.

The aetiology of glue ear is unclear but is likely to be multifactorial. A major determinant is repeated upper respiratory tract infections, making the condition more common during the winter. It is also likely that poor Eustachian tube function contributes to a predisposition to glue ear and the tendency to suffer repeated episodes of acute otitis media.

The detection of the hearing loss can be difficult and many children with the condition go undiagnosed. In the majority this is not a problem as the condition resolves spontaneously without any long term sequelae. However, it is obviously important for family practitioners to identify those patients in whom the condition persists.

History: it is vital for members of the primary health care team to listen to parents' concerns that the child is not hearing properly, and to arrange for the child's hearing to be assessed. Glue ear may present with any of the following:

- language delay
- behavioural problems
- reading/learning problems at school.

Children with glue ear are more likely to suffer from recurrent episodes of acute otitis media. Review of children with such histories, in between episodes of infection, can help identify those patients where significant middle ear effusion persists.

Examination: the appearance of the tympanic membrane in glue ear is variable and coming to a diagnosis on the basis of otoscopy alone can be difficult. The eardrum is dull and featureless (Figure 2.14), and fluid levels may be seen behind it.

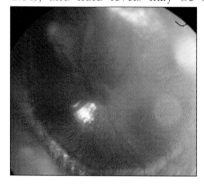

Figure 2.14 *Appearance of the left tympanic membrane in glue ear.*

Immobility of the eardrum on altering the canal pressure with a pneumatic auriscope may help make the diagnosis, although tympanometry (if available) is superior. Sometimes the eardrum is retracted towards the middle ear and may rest against the promontory or the incudo-stapedial joint.

The Rinne test should be carried out on children who are over 4 years old: in the presence of significant glue ear it is likely to be negative.

Investigation and assessment: an assessment of the hearing impairment is also important at some point. This hearing loss may fluctuate (it is often worse with colds), and is a conductive loss of about 30–35 dB. The loss tends to affect the lower frequencies (250 Hz, 500 Hz) more than the higher frequencies (Figure 2.15). This is equivalent to blocking off the ear canals with the index fingers.

Many family practitioners are able to arrange direct referral to community or hospital audiology

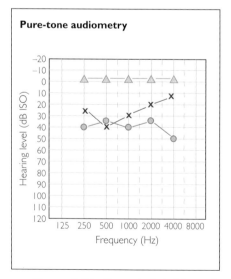

Pure-tone audiometry

Hearing level (dB ISO)

Frequency (Hz)

Figure 2.15 *Characteristic bilateral conductive hearing loss seen in glue ear.*

services. If the child is old enough to co-operate, then free field speech testing may be possible or — ideally — a pure tone audiogram can be obtained. It can be difficult to get an accurate idea of hearing thresholds, even for a paediatric audiologist. The finding of a flat tympanogram (indicating an immobile eardrum) can help confirm the diagnosis (Figure 2.16).

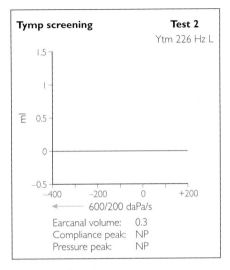

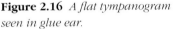

Figure 2.16 *A flat tympanogram seen in glue ear.*

If audiological assessment cannot be arranged, then it may be reasonable for family practitioners to monitor these children on the basis of the history provided by the parents, otoscopy and tuning fork tests, considering that the majority of cases will resolve spontaneously and will never require referral. Auto-inflation — by nasally blowing up a balloon via a plastic nose piece (Otovent) — is sometimes recommended in this observation period: it is cheap and does no harm. Cases which have failed to resolve after 3 months should be referred for further assessment in the ENT department.

Assessment and management of glue ear in the ENT department

There is as yet no effective medical treatment for established glue ear. An increasingly conservative approach to surgical treatment has been seen in the UK in the last few years. Unless the impairment is severe the specialist may continue a period of watchful waiting in the hope that the condition will resolve, especially if the spring and summer are approaching. In cases of unilateral glue ear surgery is unlikely to prove necessary. However, there may be a reasonable case for surgical treatment in a child with a bilateral hearing loss of about 30 dB or greater which has lasted for more than 3 months.

Grommets promote the ventilation of the middle ear rather than the drainage of fluid. They remain in place for about 12 months, after which time they are extruded spontaneously. In the right circumstances grommet insertion can produce a miraculous improvement as far as the child and the parents are concerned.

The commonest complication of grommet insertion is ear discharge, which should be treated with a combination of antibiotic and corticosteroid ear drops. Oral antibiotics are less effective.

Swimming does not influence the incidence of infection or discharge and so children are usually allowed to surface swim without taking any precautions (i.e. without having to use ear plugs).

Hearing aids: in a few cases it may be reasonable to provide children with hearing aids to help their hearing loss until such time as they 'outgrow' the problem. This option may be the most appropriate for the small number of children who have had repeated grommet insertions in the past, as they sometimes suffer grossly retracted tympanic membranes with associated hearing loss ('adhesive' otitis media).

Key points

- Childhood hearing loss needs early detection and management if adequate speech and language are to develop.
- The importance of heeding parental suspicions of hearing problems cannot be overemphasized.
- In the majority of children glue ear resolves spontaneously.
- Tympanometry is more objective than otoscopy and where available can be used to monitor the condition.
- Medical therapy does not appear to accelerate the natural resolution rate.
- There may be a reasonable case for surgical treatment in a child with a bilateral hearing loss of about 30 dB or greater which has lasted for more than 3 months.

- Children with unilateral glue ear are unlikely to require surgical treatment.

Consider referring

- Children in the at-risk groups for sensorineural hearing loss.
- Children whom the parents feel are not hearing properly.
- Bilateral glue ear that fails to resolve after 3 months.

Hearing loss in adults

A hearing loss may be sensorineural, conductive or mixed (Table 2.5). Approximately 20% of adults have a hearing impairment, the majority of cases being sensorineural and occurring in the older population. Although many patients attribute their hearing problem to wax in the ear, this is not usually the case. Unless wax is impacted it is rarely the cause of a significant hearing loss.

Table 2.5 Comparison of sensorineural and conductive hearing loss

Sensorineural hearing loss
- Results from damage to the cochlea or eighth nerve
- Aetiology is often unclear
- Will not be helped by a surgical approach and may require the help of a hearing aid

Conductive hearing loss
- Will be produced by any disease affecting the outer or middle ear
- Will be diagnosed from the history, examination and tests of hearing
- May be amenable to surgery

Diagnosis

The history may identify aetiological factors responsible for a sensorineural loss, and otoscopy will identify the majority of conditions that cause a conductive loss.

The whisper test will confirm the presence of an impairment, and tuning forks tests will indicate whether the loss is conductive or sensorineural.

Pure tone audiometry is necessary to confirm the severity and type of impairment, although the patient's level of disability may not be directly related to the pure tone audiogram. A pure tone audiogram does not give an idea of the patient's ability to 'discriminate', as speech is far more complex than pure tones.

History

How much trouble is the patient having? Often the earliest sign of an impairment is when the patient notices problems listening to conversation against a noisy background. As the hearing loss increases there will be difficulty in hearing a one-to-one conversation, in listening to the television (the patient will be accused by other members of the family of having the volume set at excessive levels) and in using the telephone.

What is the natural history of the impairment? Most problems affect both ears and are slowly progressive. However, on occasion the loss can be sudden in onset: a sudden onset sensorineural hearing loss is an emergency and the patient should be referred for an urgent opinion. Fluctuating hearing losses are less common in adults but can sometimes be related to fluctuating middle ear effusions causing a conductive loss, and in early Menière's disease the low frequency sensorineural loss can fluctuate.

Is the loss asymmetrical? The commonest reason for one ear to be worse than the other is that there is a conductive defect in the poorer ear. However, if the loss is sensorineural and asymmetrical (Figure 2.17) then the patient will require further investigation to exclude a serious cause for the asymmetry. In practice this is likely to involve an MRI scan to exclude an acoustic neuroma (Figure 2.18).

Are there any associated audiovestibular symptoms? If the patient has associated tinnitus, imbalance, otalgia or aural discharge then further investigation — and hence referral — may be indicated.

Are there any obvious aetiological factors? The following should be considered.

■ Discharge from the ears: the presence of a profuse, painless discharge suggests the presence of chronic suppurative otitis media (CSOM).

■ Risk factors for sensorineural hearing loss: a family history of deafness, exposure to noise, head injury and ototoxic drugs may all suggest a possible cause of a sensorineural loss.

■ General health: some generalized diseases are thought to have an effect on hearing, e.g. in the older age group a vascular aetiology for the loss may be suggested if the patient suffers from other vascular problems.

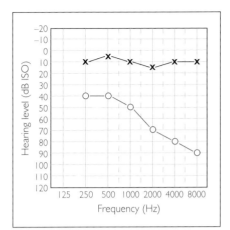

Figure 2.17 *Pure tone audiogram showing asymmetrical sensorineural hearing loss.*

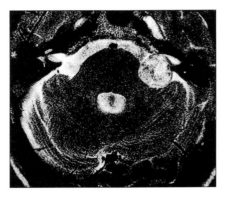

Figure 2.18 *MRI scan showing an acoustic neuroma (patient presented with an asymmetric sensorineural hearing loss).*

Examination

Lip-reading: while taking a history it may become apparent that the patient is carefully 'watching' what is said during the consultation and has in fact unknowingly taught him- or herself to lip-read.

Operation scars: their presence may suggest a history of chronic otitis media, and also that any visual abnormality of the eardrum may be related to surgery and not necessarily to a disease process. Even an ENT specialist may have problems establishing the anatomy in an operated ear!

Ear canal: if wax is present and obscuring a view of the eardrum it needs to be removed. The presence of pus or debris implies an otitis externa if the eardrum is intact, or an active chronic otitis media if there is a tympanic membrane perforation.

Eardrum and middle ear: perforations of the eardrum can occur in the absence of discharge (inactive chronic otitis media, traumatic perforations, resolving acute otitis media) and the degree of associated hearing loss will depend on the site of the perforation and the extent of associated middle ear disease (i.e. presence of erosion or fixation of the ossicular chain).

- If the eardrum is intact but has white 'chalk patches' within it (tympanosclerosis), then this and the associated hearing loss are related to the end result of some form of otitis media.
- If the eardrum is intact but immobile then the diagnosis is probably otitis media with effusion (OME, glue ear).
- If the eardrum is intact and mobile and tuning fork tests suggest a conductive loss, then the diagnosis is likely to be otosclerosis (fixation of the stapes) or, more rarely, an ossicular disruption (usually associated with a history of head injury).

Management: general

Each individual patient's management will depend on age,

lifestyle, degree of disability, type of hearing loss, its presumed aetiology and the presence of other symptoms. In general, almost all hearing impairment can be helped by a hearing aid. If there is a conductive component, surgery may also be of benefit.

Sensorineural hearing loss: causes and management

Presbyacusis is the term applied to hearing loss due to ageing. It is usually bilateral, symmetrical and the age of onset is variable. Audiometry reveals a high frequency loss. Consonants in speech are generally in the high frequencies and they are crucial for speech to be intelligible. This explains why some of these patients state that while they know that people are speaking, they cannot understand what is being said.

When a significant social handicap is present then a hearing aid may offer some hearing improvement. As a rough guide, any patient with a bilateral loss of greater than 35 dB across the frequencies may benefit from an aid.

Noise trauma: acoustic trauma occurs from sudden exposure (e.g. blast injury, gunfire) or from prolonged exposure to excessive noise. After such exposure the hearing loss may initially be reversible (a temporary threshold shift). After more prolonged exposure a permanent threshold shift occurs. The typical audiogram shows a fall in hearing at 4000 Hz.

Treatment is by avoidance or by employing adequate ear protection. In industry, noise levels of 90 dB or greater mean that the issue of ear defenders to workers is compulsory. The methods of protection are head muffs or ear plugs or both. Ear plugs offer less protection than muffs, and cotton wool in the ears is useless. A system of compensation is available for occupational hearing loss.

Ototoxic drugs: as soon as a drug is implicated as being a possible aetiological factor it should be stopped. The principal groups of drugs involved are:

- aminoglycosides
- loop diuretics such as frusemide
- salicylates
- chemotherapeutic agents such as cisplatinum.

Acoustic neuroma: this diagnosis needs to be excluded in any patient with unilateral or asymmetrical audiovestibular symptoms, including hearing loss. It is a benign tumour and is a rare cause of asymmetrical sensorineural loss (incidence is about 1 per 100,000 population per year). Although benign, if left untreated it can expand into the posterior fossa leading to potentially fatal complications from brain stem compression. It is, therefore, important to identify this tumour as early as possible and this is best achieved by an MRI scan, which is now the investigation of choice. Management will often involve surgery, although a watch and wait policy may be appropriate under certain circumstances (e.g. in the elderly), as the tumour is slow-growing and the surgery required extensive. In many hospitals surgery will be performed as a combined neurosurgical/ENT procedure.

Sudden (idiopathic) sensorineural hearing loss is a medical emergency and patients should be referred for an urgent ENT assessment. It is often difficult for the family practitioner to know that there is a significant sensorineural loss as opposed to some simple problem such as Eustachian tube dysfunction. Tuning fork tests will help in making the diagnosis but it is important to beware of a false negative Rinne test. It may be more obvious that there has been a labyrinthine upset when the hearing loss is associated with the onset of tinnitus or vertigo.

Most sudden losses are unilateral but occasionally they are bilateral. The majority will recover spontaneously but a significant number do not.

Early treatment is largely empirical, consisting of one or more of the following:

- bed rest
- vasodilators — carbogen (95% oxygen, 5% carbon dioxide) is advocated by some but requires admission to hospital
- steroids.

If recovery is going to take place, it is usually within 4–6 weeks. After the acute phase most patients would undergo an MRI scan to exclude an acoustic neuroma.

Conductive hearing loss: causes and management

Chronic otitis media without associated cholesteatoma: if there is a chronic perforation but no associated cholesteatoma, then surgery to repair the perforation (myringoplasty) is an option, although it is not essential. The main aim of surgery is to repair the defect in the eardrum to decrease the incidence of infection and to avoid the need for taking precautions when coming into contact with water, e.g. when swimming. It may also help the hearing, although there is no guarantee of this. Surgery is not 100% successful: success rates for closing the defect for most surgeons would be of the order of 70–80%.

Chronic otitis media with associated cholesteatoma: if the chronic otitis media is associated with cholesteatoma then surgery is indicated and a mastoid exploration would be required. Under these circumstances the surgery is aiming at giving a 'safe' ear which is dry (avoiding the potentially serious complications associated with a cholesteatoma). At best the hearing will stay at its current levels, but it may be worse following the surgery. However, without surgery the hearing would deteriorate in the presence of the cholesteatoma.

Otosclerosis is a disease where new bone growth occurs in the capsule of the inner ear, especially in the region of the footplate of the stapes. This may fix the stapes resulting in a conductive hearing loss. Treatment options include:

- no treatment, when the hearing loss is mild/unilateral
- hearing aids, which are often very helpful (as in most cases of conductive hearing loss) and completely safe
- stapedectomy (removing the stapes and replacing it with a piston), which may restore normal hearing but presents a small risk of total hearing loss in the operated ear.

Otitis media with effusion (OME, glue ear): many adults present complaining of dullness of hearing following an upper respiratory tract infection — a problem of Eustachian tube dysfunction. This requires no treatment other than reassurance that it will settle over a period of a few weeks.

A few patients may develop a frank middle ear effusion and again one would expect this to settle spontaneously. In these patients it would normally be a bilateral problem, although it is sometimes unilateral. If there is evidence of unilateral middle ear effusion, with typical clinical features, a negative Rinne test and persisting for 4–6 weeks, then referral is indicated to exclude any pathology within the postnasal space, e.g. nasopharyngeal carcinoma.

Key points

- Approximately 20% of adults have a hearing impairment.
- Unless wax is impacted it is rarely the cause of a significant hearing loss.
- Otoscopy should identify the common causes of a conductive loss.
- A progressive unilateral sensorineural hearing loss should be fully investigated to exclude an acoustic neuroma.
- In general, sensorineural losses are managed by amplification.
- Conductive hearing losses can be managed by amplification, surgery or both.

Consider referring

- Patients with unilateral sensorineural hearing loss (to exclude an acoustic neuroma).
- Patients with bilateral loss of greater than 35 dB across the frequencies who may benefit from a hearing aid.
- Patients with hearing loss and other associated audiovestibular symptoms such as vertigo, otalgia or aural discharge.
- Conductive hearing loss where surgery may help, e.g. otosclerosis, ossicular disruption.
- Sudden onset sensorineural hearing loss should be referred as an emergency.
- Chronic otitis media where associated cholesteatoma is suspected.
- Stable chronic otitis media for closure of the eardrum perforation to reduce the incidence of infection.
- Persisting unilateral middle ear effusion (glue ear) to exclude postnasal space pathology.

Aids to hearing

Hearing loss is a major disability that can interfere with the patient's work, education and social life. A bilateral hearing loss of 35 dB or more in the speech frequency range 500–3000 Hz can result in significant problems that may be helped by one or more of the following remedies:

- hearing aids
- environmental aids
- lip-reading/sign language
- cochlear implants.

Hearing aids

In the UK, over 200,000 hearing aids are issued by the NHS each year. In view of the projected increase in the elderly population these figures are set to rise significantly, and family practitioners will be questioned increasingly about hearing aids by their patients.

Presbyacusis: most of the patients who enquire about the benefits of a hearing aid will be older patients suffering from varying degrees of presbyacusis. If an audiogram is available and their hearing thresholds across the frequencies are better than 30–35 dB, it is unlikely that they will be helped significantly. However, if the patient seems to be having increasing problems then it may be reasonable to opt for a therapeutic trial with an aid, whatever the audiogram thresholds.

In general, the poorer the patient's hearing is, the greater the benefit and the more likely he or she is to use the aid. It is desirable for elderly patients suffering from presbyacusis to be referred relatively early, before more severe deafness and infirmity make it difficult for them to cope with the skills required to use a hearing aid correctly.

Using a hearing aid is not as simple as wearing glasses. Inserting the mould can be difficult to master, and the aid needs to be switched on and the volume set. In order for patients to gain the maximum benefit, it is important that they are given appropriate training and that follow-up is provided within the audiology department to ensure that they are not having any difficulties. If such support is not provided many aids remain in a drawer!

Conductive deafness: it is worth remembering that patients with conductive deafness find hearing aids extremely helpful so that their use should be considered in otosclerosis or patients with middle ear effusions (glue ear).

Hearing aid problems: hearing aids can malfunction mechanically. The most common problem is acoustic feedback (producing the familiar high-pitched whistle), which is more likely to occur:
- if the patient requires high amplification
- if the patient has a poor fitting mould

- if the plastic tube is blocked (patients are instructed to change the tube every 2 months and are given a supply of replacements).

Chronic irritation and discharge caused by an aid may be helped by fitting a perforated mould, or by changing the material of the mould if an allergic reaction is suspected.

Choosing which ear(s) to fit: in general, when there is a mild or moderate impairment a monaural aid is fitted to the poorer ear. If there is a severe impairment a monaural aid is fitted to the better ear. Binaural aids often are difficult to manage and are reserved for the more severely disabled.

Parts of an electronic air conduction hearing aid

- Microphone, which picks up incoming sound.
- Amplifier, which makes the sound louder and is adjustable.
- Mould, which is worn in the ear canal and delivers the sound to the ear (in bone conduction aids the sound is delivered by a vibrator on the skull). A mould is cast from an impression of the outer ear canal and concha taken with a rapidly setting plastic material.
- Volume control.
- OTM switch, where O is for off, M for microphone on, and T is for switching the microphone to the telecoil that allows the use of electromagnetic induction waves to provide sound and cut out background noise (induction loop system).

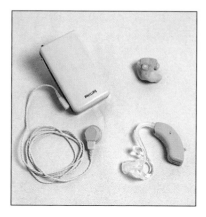

Figure 2.19 *Different types of hearing aid, which include: body worn (BW) aid (left); behind the ear (BE) aid (bottom right); in the ear (IE) aid (top right).*

Types of hearing aid available
(Figure 2.19)

- *Behind the ear (BE) aids* are the commonest type of aid prescribed within the NHS and are sufficiently powerful for all but the profoundly impaired.
- *'In the ear' and 'in the canal' aids* are accommodated entirely in the external ear and are only suitable for those with mild or moderate impairment. Some are in theory available through the NHS, but in practice lack of funding often means that they are not provided.
- *Body worn aids* are rarely prescribed but may be necessary for patients with profound hearing loss (these aids are more powerful) or patients who do not have the manipulative skills required to use a small BE aid.
- *Bone conduction aids* are only occasionally necessary when a conventional ear mould cannot be used, e.g. a chronically infected, discharging ear or atresia of the ear canal. Traditionally the bone conductor vibrator is held onto the mastoid by a headband, but more recently osseointegrated bone-anchored aids have been used.

Obtaining hearing aids

Direct referral to an audiology department: most of the patients to be fitted with a hearing aid will be adults with a bilateral symmetric sensorineural hearing loss, idiopathic in origin but age-related. For this group a specialist medical opinion is probably unnecessary in the absence of other otologic symptoms. In some areas a direct referral system is available whereby the family practitioner refers the patient direct to the hearing aid department without an ENT assessment being included.

The following guidelines should be followed for direct referral.

- Patient aged 60 years or over.
- Patient must have been seen by a family practitioner and had his or her ears dewaxed.
- There should be no other otologic symptoms.
- The eardrums should look normal and not be perforated.
- The Rinne tests should be positive and the Weber central, i.e. no evidence of conductive deafness and no asymmetric hearing loss.

Referral to an ENT specialist: the main role of the ENT specialist is screening:

- to exclude other symptoms
- to look in the ears to detect conductive causes (i.e. surgically treatable causes) for the hearing loss
- to arrange further investigation for any patients with asymmetric audiovestibular symptoms.

Private dispensers: the patient does not need initial referral by a family practitioner to obtain an aid. A wider selection of aids is available commercially (many patients resort to this sector to purchase a cosmetically acceptable in the ear hearing aid) but they can be expensive. Many private dispensers provide patients with binaural aids, as opposed to the practice within the NHS, where they are reserved for the more severely disabled.

Environmental aids

Many products are available that may assist the deaf patient in routine daily life.

- Doorbells and telephone bells may be changed to lower tones (buzzers), louder volumes or flashing lights.
- Telephones can be fitted with volume controls and can be converted for use with the telecoil induction switch in a hearing aid.
- Televisions may have a direct output to headphones or use an induction loop system (one model has a loop of wire from the television to a cushion that is placed on the seat where the user sits).
- Induction loop systems for those using hearing aids are available in many theatres, churches, etc., and can be used with televisions and telephones if these are modified. Loops can also be installed in nursing homes for the elderly, providing great benefit to the large proportion of residents who wear hearing aids.

Lip-reading/sign language

Most patients with hearing loss will benefit from the development of lip-reading skills (indeed, many patients unknowingly acquire the skill). However, if at all possible normal speech and language development in children with severe hearing loss should be encouraged by amplification of any residual hearing. Manual communication skills using sign language can only be used with others who have similar skills.

Cochlear implants

A cochlear implant ('bionic ear') is a device used in patients with a non-functioning cochlea but who have a normal cochlear nerve. They are only appropriate for the profoundly or totally bilaterally deaf who obtain no benefit from conventional aids.

The system consists of an ear-level microphone which collects sound, and a body-worn speech processor to convert the sound to electrical signals. These signals are then passed to an electrode that has been fed through the turns of the cochlea at the time of the surgery, and thus stimulate the cochlear nerve directly, bypassing the cochlea (Figure 2.20). The cochlear nerve stimulation gives clues to cadences and frequencies, and is an aid to lip reading. As these devices have improved (in terms of the speech processing), so they have afforded better speech perception, with some patients being able to use a telephone.

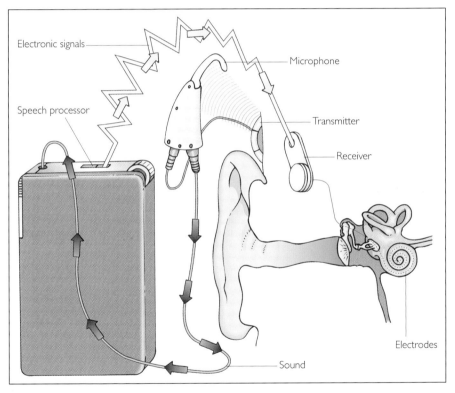

Figure 2.20 *A diagram to show the constituents of the cochlear implant system.*

Key points

- Hearing aids do not produce normal hearing.
- If hearing thresholds across the frequencies are better than 30–35 dB, then it is unlikely that the patient will be helped by a hearing aid.
- Hearing aids can be of considerable benefit and nothing is lost by trying one out.
- Behind the ear (BE) aids are the commonest type of aid prescribed within the NHS and are sufficiently powerful for all but the profoundly impaired.
- Patients referred by the family practitioner direct to the audiology department for a hearing aid should be over 60, have normal eardrums and tuning fork tests, and have no other otologic symptoms.

Consider referring

- Patients with bilateral hearing loss of greater than 35 dB across the frequencies.
- Patients with presbyacusis with a milder hearing loss but who are having increasing problems (for a therapeutic trial of an aid).
- Patients with conductive deafness caused by otosclerosis or glue ear.

The dizzy patient

'There can be few physicians so dedicated to their art that they do not experience a slight decline in spirits on learning that their patient's complaint is giddiness.'   (Matthews, 1970)

Table 2.6 Non-otological and otological causes of dizziness

Non-otological causes

- Drugs
- Cervical spondylosis
- Postural hypotension
- Transient ischaemic attacks
- Cerebrovascular disease
- Vertebrobasilar ischaemia
- Migraine
- Anxiety/hyperventilation (dizzy spells are a discriminant on the Goldberg scale for measuring anxiety)
- Multiple sclerosis

Otological causes

- Benign paroxysmal positional vertigo BPPV
- Labyrinthitis/vestibular neuronitis/acute labyrinthine failure
- Menière's disease
- Acoustic neuroma
- Chronic suppurative otitis media (CSOM) with cholesteatoma
- Trauma to inner ear
- Rupture of round or oval window

A family practitioner with 2000 patients can expect to see approximately 30 patients each year presenting with disturbance of balance as a new symptom and the main reason for the consultation. Many more patients will complain of giddiness as part of their presenting illness, and dizziness is reported by about 30% of people over 65 years of age. The causes of dizziness may be otological or non-otological (Table 2.6).

In family practice most patients complaining of giddiness describe light-headed, faint feelings rather than true rotational vertigo, and history-taking and examination will be directed towards identifying a non-vestibular cause. Where the patient describes rotational vertigo or other sensations of disorientation in space, the main task is to identify the site of the defect — the pathology may be peripheral (otological) or central (brain stem) — and, if possible, to define its aetiology.

Where dizziness is concerned, investigations are often of minimal benefit in arriving at a diagnosis (indeed, in many patients *no one* will make a diagnosis): the history is the key.

Physiology of the vestibular system (Figure 2.21): the brain stem acts as the co-ordinating centre and receives input from the eyes, limbs and vestibular system of the ear. The cerebellum co-ordinates body movements in response to these sensory inputs, and the cerebrum also has an influence in the response. Provide a faulty or contradictory input from any one of the 'inputs' and dizziness occurs.

History

In patients with dizziness, the history is the key to diagnosis.

Is the dizziness associated with a loss of consciousness? If the patient has an altered state of consciousness or loses consciousness, then the problem is likely to be central.

What is the natural history of the severity? Central causes of imbalance are usually progressive. However, the first episode of otological dizziness tends to be the worst; subsequent episodes tend to be less severe as the system compensates.

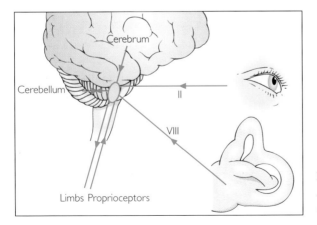

Figure 2.21
Physiology of the vestibular system.

Is there a precipitating factor such as position? If the episodes are brought on by certain head movements (e.g. on lying down or turning over in bed at night) and last for a short period (for seconds up to a minute), then the diagnosis is likely to be benign paroxysmal positional vertigo (BPPV).

What is the duration of the dizziness? In BPPV the vertigo lasts for seconds, in Menière's disease for 30 minutes to 12 hours, and in acute labyrinthine failure it can last for days to weeks.

Are there any otological symptoms during the episodes? The presence of auditory symptoms such as hearing loss or tinnitus (which is especially significant if it is unilateral) supports a peripheral labyrinthine cause for the dizziness.

Are there any associated symptoms?
- Nausea and vomiting are typical accompaniments of labyrinthine dizziness.
- Central causes of dizziness (e.g. vertebrobasilar insufficiency, multiple sclerosis) are associated with other neurological symptoms (e.g. dysarthria, visual disturbance).
- Cerebellar lesions tend to cause ataxia only, with no vertigo or nystagmus unless the vestibular connections are involved.

What drugs is the patient taking? Almost any drug can cause imbalance.

Examination in general practice
Otoscopy: the tympanic membranes should be examined for evidence of middle ear disease, in particular cholesteatoma, which can erode the labyrinth.

Hearing assessment: tuning fork tests and audiology should be used to identify unilateral hearing loss. If present, exclusion of an acoustic neuroma is mandatory.

Cardiovascular assessment: lying/standing blood pressure, pulse and carotid bruits should be assessed.

Neurological assessment: the cranial nerves, gait and co-ordination should be assessed. Dorsal column problems should be excluded using the Romberg test.

The Unterberger test is a useful test of the vestibular system. The patient is asked to stretch the arms out in front with the fingers separated whilst walking on the spot: this saturates the proprioceptive pathways. The eyes should be closed, thereby removing ocular fixation. This effectively leaves only vestibular input into the balance pathways. If the patient is able to maintain his or her balance, then the vestibular system is probably intact.

Nystagmus: this is a repetitious slow drift of the eyes in one direction with a rapid correction back to the starting point (by convention the direction of the nystagmus is the direction of the fast correction component). The characteristics of the nystagmus can help to differentiate between central neurological and peripheral vestibular causes of vertigo (Table 2.7).

Positional testing for nystagmus (the Hallpike test) is useful in patients with BPPV. The patient is asked to sit on an examination couch and the head is suddenly put backwards to just below the

---

Table 2.7 Comparison of peripheral-type and central-type nystagmus

Peripheral-type nystagmus	Central-type nystagmus
■ Horizontal/rotatory	■ Vertical
■ Never vertical	■ Changes direction
■ Same in both eyes	■ May be different in the two eyes
■ Fast component usually away from diseased ear	

level of the couch (Figure 2.22). In BPPV nystagmus is induced when the affected ear is lowermost, coming on after about 5–10 seconds and lasting up to 40 seconds.

Examination and assessment in the ENT department
It should be remembered that, despite assessment in both ENT and neurology departments, a large number of patients suffering from dizziness will still not be given a specific diagnosis.

Pure tone audiograms: all dizzy patients attending an ENT clinic should undergo a pure tone audiogram to identify any who have a significant asymmetrical sensorineural hearing loss.

MRI scans: if a significant asymmetrical sensorineural hearing loss is identified, the patient should be referred for an MRI scan to exclude the possibility of an acoustic neuroma as the cause of the symptoms.

Caloric tests: if the audiogram identified no asymmetry then it might be reasonable to arrange caloric tests. If normal, it would suggest that the peripheral vestibular function is normal: if the symptoms

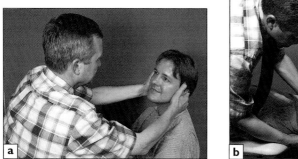
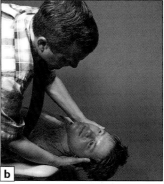

Figure 2.22 *Positional testing is useful in patients with benign paroxysmal positional vertigo. (a) Staring position. (b) Patient head dropped below the level of the couch and rotated to one side.*

69

persist then a neurological opinion might be appropriate to exclude a central cause. If the caloric test identified a canal paresis then again this would prompt an MRI scan to exclude an acoustic neuroma.

Nystagmus induced by peripheral lesions is enhanced in the dark and diminished by occular fixation. Electronystagmography and Frenzel's glasses (powerful magnifying glasses) will respectively overcome these difficulties and allow a more accurate assessment of the nystagmus.

Table 2.8 Peripheral and central vertigo

Benign paroxysmal positional vertigo (BPPV)
- Latent period
- Fatigue on repetition
- Vertiginous during test
- Peripheral-type nystagmus

Central positional vertigo
- Immediate onset
- No fatigue on repetition
- Often asymptomatic

Benign paroxysmal positional vertigo (BPPV)

This is the commonest cause of episodic vertigo in family practice. It should be differentiated from central positional vertigo (Table 2.8). Symptoms of BPPV include:

- precipitated by sudden change in position, e.g. lying down or turning over in bed
- peripheral-type nystagmus after latent period of about 10 seconds
- short-lived nystagmus (usually less than 60 seconds)
- associated nausea usually
- responses become less prominent, or fatigue is shown on repetition
- no auditory symptoms
- positional testing pathognomonic.

Almost all cases of BPPV can be managed in family practice and referral for further investigation is only necessary if the course of the illness is atypical. Recovery usually occurs over 3–6 months; treatment is with short courses of labyrinthine sedatives and vestibular exercises.

Labyrinthitis/vestibular neuronitis/acute labyrinthine failure

Symptoms include:

- sudden onset of prostrating vertigo with profuse vomiting
- nystagmus usually present for first 24–48 hours
- hearing loss is not a feature
- adaptation occurs in 10 days to 3 weeks, but even then vertigo may return in the dark with loss of ocular fixation.

Treatment is with parenteral sedatives initially, and then with oral labyrinthine sedatives. Referral is not required unless there is a suspicion of hearing loss.

Menière's disease (endolymphatic hydrops)

Menière's disease, which is relatively rare in family practice, is the result of an increase in endolymphatic pressure in the labyrinth, although what causes this is unclear. Symptoms include:

- episodic vertigo — intermittent attacks of severe vertigo and vomiting lasting from 15 min-utes to 12 hours
- episodes are usually preceded by (or associated with) tin-nitus, a sense of fullness in the ear, sound distortion and fluctuating hearing loss (usually unilateral)
- may be long periods (months) between attacks
- hearing loss in lower frequencies initially and sensorineural in type (Figure 2.23)
- later in the disease higher frequencies also affected
- after each episode a little

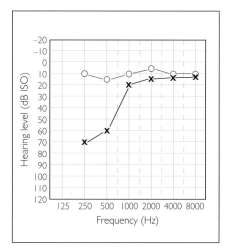

Figure 2.23 *Characteristic pure tone audiogram in a patient with left sided Menière's disease in the early stages (note the low frequency sensorineural hearing loss).*

71

more hearing is lost, and eventually hearing in the affected ear may be totally lost

■ in the majority of cases the condition is unilateral but progresses to involve the other ear in up to 20% of patients.

Initial management is usually undertaken by the family practictioner: an acute attack may require intramuscular, buccal or rectal prochlorperazine. Prophylaxis is a controversial area, but betahistine (16 mg tds) together with a vestibular sedative (cinnarizine 15 mg tds) may be a reasonable combination.

Referral: the patient often develops unilateral sensorineural hearing loss as the condition progresses. Referral for an MRI scan to exclude an acoustic neuroma is then advisable. Unilateral tinnitus would also require an MRI scan.

The natural history is for the condition to resolve (apart from the hearing loss), but for a small minority of patients surgery may provide the only solution. Surgical treatments involve hearing-conservation procedures (e.g. decompression of the endolymphatic sac, division of the vestibular nerve) or procedures which sacrifice hearing in that ear (labyrinthectomy).

Acoustic neuroma

The incidence of acoustic neuroma is approximately 1 per 100,000 population per year. These benign tumours arise from the audiovestibular nerve within the internal auditory canal and initially produce only audiovestibular symptoms (unilateral hearing loss or tinnitus). As a neuroma expands it may cause other cranial neuropathies (affecting trigeminal, facial and vagal group), brain stem compression and raised intracranial pressure. Vertigo occurs late in the course of the illness as central adaptation occurs because the tumour is slow growing.

As early diagnosis is crucial, it is important for family practitioners to maintain a high index of suspicion in patients with unilateral audiovestibular symptoms: mortality and morbidity from surgery is directly related to tumour size. It is particularly important to beware of a false negative Rinne test.

Other otological causes of dizziness

Chronic suppurative otitis media (CSOM) with cholesteatoma may cause erosion of the labyrinth and hence a fistula between the middle and inner ear.

Trauma to the inner ear: surgical trauma, head injury with associated temporal bone fracture, and barotrauma may all result in dizziness.

Rupture of the round or the oval window produces sudden onset of unilateral hearing loss and tinnitus, and vertigo. Symptoms usually occur after sudden changes in pressure, e.g. during air travel or during sudden exercise. Early referral to hospital for repair is essential.

Key points

- The history is the key to diagnosis.
- The site of the defect should be identified: the pathology may be peripheral (otological) or central (brain stem).
- Imbalance which lasts for 1–2 seconds only is of no clinical significance.
- Investigations are often of minimal benefit in arriving at a diagnosis.
- Hearing assessment is required to identify unilateral hearing loss. If present, exclusion of an acoustic neuroma is mandatory.
- Unilateral tinnitus requires exclusion of an acoustic neuroma.
- In a large number of patients no diagnosis will be made.
- Management when no specific cause is found includes reassurance that things are likely to improve, vestibular

sedatives (e.g. antihistamines, phenothiazines, anticholinergics) and vestibular exercises (to encourage process of adaptation).

■ Most patients with giddiness can be managed by family practitioners.

Consider referring

■ Atypical cases of BPPV, e.g. lasting longer than 6 months.
■ Acute labyrinthitis/vestibular neuronitis/acute labyrinthine failure if there is any suspicion of hearing loss.
■ Menière's disease, which may present with associated unilateral sensorineural hearing loss and/or unilateral tinnitus requiring an MRI scan to exclude acoustic neuroma.
■ Any patient with vertigo and unilateral sensorineural hearing loss.
■ Any patient with known CSOM who develops vertigo (cholesteatoma may cause erosion of the labyrinth).

Tinnitus

Noises in the ear are called tinnitus and it is therefore a symptom as opposed to a diagnosis. It is extremely common (affecting about 15% of the population at some time or other) and can be extremely alarming, especially in the first few weeks following its onset. Fortunately, in the vast majority of patients a process of adaptation occurs and the tinnitus becomes increasingly less obtrusive as time goes on. Patients can therefore be reassured at the onset of their tinnitus that it is a common problem and does not signify the presence of some underlying sinister pathology.

There are two types of tinnitus:

■ otologic (subjective) tinnitus, which only the patient can hear, is by far the most common and is usually ascribed to some form of cochlear abnormality

■ transmitted (objective) tinnitus can sometimes be heard by the doctor as well as the patient.

Otologic (subjective) tinnitus

This is often likened to a high-pitched hiss and is not usually pulsatile. The severity of the tinnitus varies from day to day and is often at its worst in the first few weeks following its onset. It is usually described as being at its worst in quiet surroundings and so can be particularly troublesome when the patient is trying to get to sleep. Otologic tinnitus is usually associated with some form of hearing loss but this may or may not have been noticed by the patient. It is worth remembering that many drugs can cause or exacerbate tinnitus (Table 2.9).

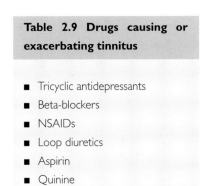

Table 2.9 Drugs causing or exacerbating tinnitus

■ Tricyclic antidepressants
■ Beta-blockers
■ NSAIDs
■ Loop diuretics
■ Aspirin
■ Quinine

Presbyacusis: in family practice by far the commonest cause of otologic tinnitus is presbyacusis with the following characteristics:

■ tinnitus is usually bilateral (or the patient may describe it as being 'inside the head')
■ normal tuning fork tests
■ normal findings on otoscopy
■ audiology shows symmetrical sensorineural hearing loss.

Patients meeting these criteria (i.e. the majority of patients seen with tinnitus in family practice) do not require referral to an ENT specialist, although some may benefit from a hearing aid referral.

Examinations and referrals: all patients presenting with tinnitus require otoscopy and audiology. Any patients noted to have an asymmetric hearing loss in association with their tinnitus require referral for further investigation to exclude any underlying pathology such as an acoustic neuroma. For the same reason any patient with unilateral tinnitus which persists for more than a few months should be referred.

Management: once underlying disease (Table 2.10) has been excluded, patient counselling is the most important aspect of management. The majority of patients adjust well to their tinnitus once they have been reassured. In the small number of patients who do not adjust there is no specific medical or surgical treatment. In these patients one or more of the following may be useful.

- A hearing aid may help those with a hearing impairment — the tinnitus is masked by the improvement in hearing.
- Masking strategies (e.g. using background music from a radio) can be used whenever it is quiet. If getting off to sleep is a problem then a clock radio can be timed to be on for an hour while the patient is trying to get to sleep.
- Tinnitus maskers look like an ear-level hearing aid but produce a background noise which many patients find to be of considerable psychological support. The rationale for such an approach is to use an extraneous noise to drown out or mask the noise of the tinnitus.

Table 2.10 Ear diseases associated with subjective tinnitus

External ear	Inner ear
■ Wax	■ Noise-induced hearing loss
	■ Presbyacusis
Middle ear	■ Menière's disease
■ Otosclerosis	■ Trauma (surgery, head injury)
■ Middle ear effusion	■ Labyrinthitis
	■ Acoustic neuroma

- Referral to a self-help and support group such as the Tinnitus Association.
- Occasionally patients may require intermittent short courses of night sedation.

Transmitted (objective) tinnitus

This type of tinnitus arises because the ear picks up sounds such as the patient's own pulse or the involuntary twitching of the muscles of the soft palate (palatal myoclonus). The majority of patients with this type of tinnitus will describe a beating quality to the sound (pulsatile tinnitus). The pulse is frequently heard in:

- conductive hearing loss
- acute inflammatory conditions affecting the ear
- vascular abnormalities, e.g. arteriovenous fistula, glomus jugulare tumours, transmitted noise from the carotid artery
- anxiety.

Transmitted tinnitus is often unilateral, so referral is often necessary to exclude underlying pathology.

Key points

- Tinnitus affects about 15% of the population.
- In the vast majority of patients seen in family practice tinnitus is caused by prebyacusis and there is no serious pathology. Once reassured, the majority of these patients will learn to cope with their tinnitus.
- Unilateral tinnitus needs full investigation.
- Pulsatile tinnitus (unless associated with an acute inflammatory problem) should be fully investigated.

Consider referring

- Any patient with unilateral tinnitus which persists for more than a few months.
- Any patient with asymmetric hearing loss in association with tinnitus.
- Patients with pulsatile tinnitus (unless associated with an acute inflammatory problem).
- Patients suffering from presbyacusis who may benefit from a hearing aid.

Facial palsy

The facial nerve

The facial nerve may be considered to have intracranial, intratemporal and extratemporal parts to its course (Figure 2.24).

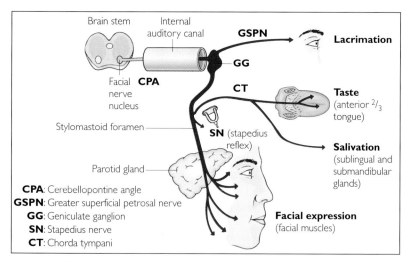

Figure 2.24 *Anatomy of the facial nerve.*

Intracranial: the cell bodies lie in the facial nuclei of the brain stem. The nerve leaves the brain stem in the cerebello-pontine angle and enters the internal auditory canal along with the cochleo-vestibular nerve.

Intratemporal: it then enters the temporal bone and takes a complex z-shaped course through it (passing through the middle ear and mastoid) to emerge through the skull base at the stylomastoid foramen.

Extratemporal: it divides into several branches whilst running through the parotid gland and goes on to supply the muscles of facial expression. Within the temporal bone the facial nerve has three branches.

Superficial petrosal nerve: this arises from the geniculate ganglion in the petrous temporal bone and carries secretomotor fibres to the lacrimal gland.

Chorda tympani: this joins the facial nerve just before it leaves the temporal bone above the stylomastoid foramen, and conveys taste from the anterior two-thirds of the tongue (via the lingual nerve).

Stapedial nerve: this arises just above the chorda tympani and supplies motor fibres to stapedius muscle.

Assessing facial palsy

The facial nerve can be affected in any part of its course and the family practitioner's assessment (Figure 2.25) should answer the following questions.

Is it an upper or lower motor neurone lesion? It is essential to differentiate an upper motor neurone (UMN) lesion from a lower motor neurone (LMN) lesion. A complete facial palsy which spares the forehead is an UMN lesion, whereas a complete LMN lesion affects all areas of the affected side of the face (Figure 2.26).

79

The commonest cause of an UMN lesion is a cerebrovascular accident, and the commonest cause of a LMN lesion is idiopathic (Bell's) palsy. However, Bell's palsy is a diagnosis made by exclusion of other causes (Table 2.11).

Are there any other associated neurological symptoms and signs? If present, these may suggest a primary cause for the facial palsy, e.g. brain stem neoplasia, brain stem infarction or a cerebellopontine angle lesion. A lesion in the brain stem, for example, might cause diplopia due to associated palsy of the sixth nerve.

Is the facial palsy complete or incomplete? If incomplete:
- neuropraxia may be assumed
- prognosis regarding recovery is better (depending on aetiology)
- it is less likely that surgical intervention will be required.

Noting the degree of paralysis is important in assessing recovery of function over the following weeks/months.

Has there been recent trauma to head, ear or face? Any trauma (including surgery) in these areas can produce a LMN facial palsy, and such cases clearly require referral.

Temporal bone fractures are usually only seen in cases of severe head injury.

If the palsy was *complete* and *immediate* in onset, there would be a case for surgical intervention. If *incomplete* and *delayed* in onset, then an expectant approach would be adopted.

Is the ear normal? If the patient has a history of otorrhoea then chronic otitis media with an associated cholesteatoma should be excluded.

A full examination of the ear is essential. All wax and debris must be removed to allow a complete examination of the auditory canal and eardrum: if this is not possible, then referral for aural toilet and examination under the microscope is indicated.

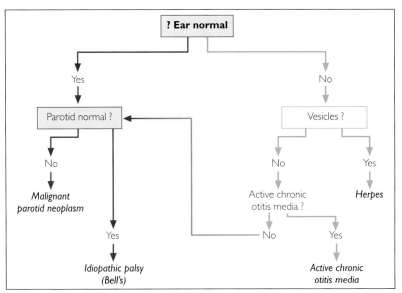

Figure 2.25 *Flow chart for assessment of facial palsy.*

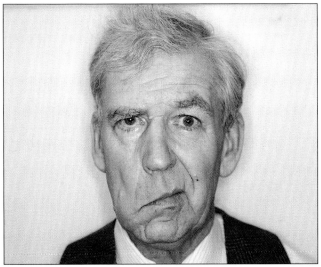

Figure 2.26 *A patient with facial nerve paralysis.*

Table 2.11 Causes of lower motor neurone (LMN) facial palsy

Intracanial
- Pons – tumours, vascular accidents
- Cerebello-pontine angle – tumours
- Internal auditory meatus – trauma, tumours

Intratemporal
- Bell's palsy
- Acute or chronic ear disease
- Herpes zoster oticus
- Temporal bone fractures
- Post-surgery
- Tumours of temporal bone

Extratemporal
- Parotid tumours
- Facial lacerations

If there is a history of hearing loss, or if abnormalities are found on the tuning fork tests, then a pure tone audiogram is necessary. If an associated hearing loss is confirmed then further investigation with CT or MRI may be indicated to exclude pathology involving the nerve in its intracranial and intratemporal course.

If there was preceding otalgia and vesicles are seen in the external ear canal, then the diagnosis is herpes zoster oticus (Ramsay Hunt syndrome).

Is the parotid gland normal? A malignant parotid tumour may be palpable in the face or neck (benign tumours rarely, if ever, involve the facial nerve). The oropharynx must be examined, as the only evidence of a deep lobe tumour may be the fact that the tonsil has been pushed medially towards the midline.

Bell's palsy

Bell's palsy (idiopathic facial paralysis) is the commonest cause of facial paralysis and is a diagnosis of exclusion.

Degree of paralysis: this should be assessed.

■ Incomplete paralysis (neuropraxia) occurs in 75% of cases. Full recovery of nerve function will happen in 3–4 weeks in 85–90% of these patients, and referral is seldom necessary.

■ Complete paralysis occurs in 25% of cases. Approximately half of these patients will show slow and incomplete recovery.

Management: drug treatment options are:

■ oral prednisolone (although there is little hard scientific evidence to support their use, a course of oral steroids is often used in cases of complete paralysis of under 7 days duration).

■ oral aciclovir has been advocated by some on the assumption of a viral cause.

Protection of the cornea and care of the eye are the most important considerations, as conjunctival infection and corneal trauma can occur because of the absence of protective blinking. In order to reduce these risks:

■ regular eyedrops (e.g. hypromellose) for lubrication should be prescribed

■ suggest the patient tapes the eye closed at night if there is incomplete closure

■ spectacles with a side protector can be used.

An ophthalmic opinion should be sought at an early stage, as a lateral tarsorrhaphy may facilitate corneal protection whilst awaiting recovery of the facial palsy.

Referral: if there is no recovery in 6 weeks then referral is advisable. The ENT specialist may:

■ confirm that there is no primary cause for the palsy by carrying out further investigations, e.g. audiology, CT or MRI scans

■ arrange electrophysiological tests to assess whether there is nerve degeneration and so give some indication of the prognosis for recovery

- involve plastic surgery colleagues who have surgical techniques available to improve facial appearance when at rest.

Key points

- Facial palsy should be presumed to originate within the ear or parotid until proven otherwise.
- Otoscopy should always be performed.
- Bell's palsy is a diagnosis of exclusion.
- Protection of the cornea is the most important factor in the early management of facial paralysis.
- 90% of cases of Bell's palsy with incomplete paralysis will recover fully in 3–4 weeks.

Consider referring

- Patients with complete Bell's palsy where there is no recovery within 6 weeks.
- Patients with other associated neurological symptoms or signs.
- Facial palsy associated with trauma.
- If a complete view of the eardrum cannot be obtained.
- If there is an associated and asymmetrical hearing loss.
- If there is an abnormality in the parotid gland.
- Patients requiring lateral tarsorrhaphy for eye protection.

Chapter 3

The nose

Epistaxis

A nose bleed — even a trivial one — can be a frightening experience for the patient. They may present either because they are actively bleeding or because they have a history of recurrent epistaxes but for the moment the bleeding has ceased. Epistaxis may have either a local or a general cause.

Local causes

Little's area (Figure 3.1): spontaneous bleeding may come from Little's area (anterior nasal septum) where there is an anastomosis of vessels from both the internal and external carotid arteries. This is by far the most common site of bleeding in children. Adults may bleed from this site, but more often will bleed from a more posterior site.

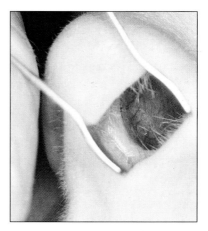

Figure 3.1 *Little's area of the nasal septum.*

Trauma: epistaxis may follow trauma such as facial injuries and nose-picking.

Neoplasms may present with epistaxis, although the bleeding is more likely to be scanty and associated with other symptoms (nasal obstruction, epiphora, facial pain).

Angiofibroma is a benign but locally invasive tumour arising near the nasopharynx, almost exclusively in adolescent males. It is highly vascular and is a rare cause of a profuse epistaxis.

General causes

Epistaxis may be associated with the following:

- hypertension
- blood dyscrasias
- anticoagulants
- anti-platelet drugs, e.g. aspirin (even in the low dose regime used in ischaemic heart disease patients)
- NSAIDs.

Managing active bleeding

When examining the patient it is obviously wise to adopt the same precautions used when dealing with any body fluids, i.e. wearing gloves, gown and possibly eye protectors. Initial treatment is aimed at controlling the haemorrhage, and the techniques employed for this will depend to some extent on whether it is an anterior or posterior bleed.

Anterior bleed: for an anterior bleed the patient's nostrils should be pinched together tightly for 10–15 minutes while breathing continues through the mouth. (It is useless to press on the bony bridge of the nose as patients often do.) The patient should sit upright and hold a bowl to spit out any clots that run down the nasopharynx.

This first aid measure can normally be expected to stop bleeding from this site. However, if the bleeding does continue (or if the bleeding point can be identified) then an attempt should be made to *cauterize* the nose. The nose should be anaesthetized (cotton wool soaked in 5% cocaine or 4% lignocaine can be placed in the anterior nares for 5 minutes) and the bleeding point then cauterized with a silver nitrate stick (Figure 3.2). This manoeuvre is very uncomfortable and so should not be attempted without local anaesthesia.

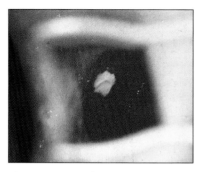

Figure 3.2 *Anterior nasal septum after cautery with silver nitrate.*

Persisting active bleeding: it is usually very difficult to establish either an exact cause or the site of the bleed (although it can be assumed to be anterior in almost all children), and an anterior nasal pack may be required. The traditional method is to pack the nose with ribbon gauze soaked in bismuth iodoform paraffin paste (BIPP). More modern alternatives are inflatable balloon catheters of various designs and, more recently, a Merocel pack (Figure 3.3) that expands when saline is dripped onto it and which may be an easier alternative.

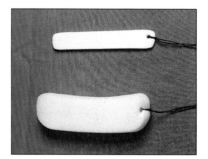

Figure 3.3 *Merocel nasal pack before and after the addition of 5–10 ml of saline.*

Posterior bleeding: in most adults, particularly the elderly, epistaxes arise from a posterior site. Since the bleeding point is usually neither visible nor accessible to cautery, initial treatment involves some form of tamponade using an anterior nasal pack. A Merocel pack may again be the simplest alternative. Posterior bleeds may not be controlled by an anterior nasal pack, and so may require referral.

Recurrent epistaxes

In the more relaxed situation where the patient is not actively bleeding, it is possible carefully to examine the nose to try to identify the source of the bleeds. If the bleeds arise from Little's area (anterior nasal septum), then the area can be cauterized under local anaesthesia using a silver nitrate stick.

Referral is appropriate for the older group of patients in whom no anterior source can be identified, especially if there are other associated symptoms such as nasal obstruction or facial pain. In the ENT department the nose and postnasal space can be carefully examined with a nasal endoscope.

Management in the ENT department

Anterior bleeding may be more effectively dealt with using electrocautery, especially in the presence of profuse bleeding.

Continuing posterior epistaxis: management will continue within the ENT department. It may be necessary to try to seal off the posterior choana, which can be done with a Foley urethral catheter passed into the nasopharynx via the nose. The inflated balloon blocks off the posterior choana and the anterior nose is then packed with ribbon gauze. Once successfully packed, the patient is put on bed rest. These measures will usually control the bleeding, although in a small number of cases the packing may need to be done under a general anaesthetic, or the following feeding vessels may need to ligated:

■ external carotid artery in the neck
■ maxillary artery behind the posterior wall of the maxillary antrum
■ ethmoidal vessels on the medial wall of the orbit.

Key points

■ Almost all epistaxes in children arise from Little's area.
■ Most epistaxes in adults arise from a posterior source.

- Nose bleeds may be caused by aspirin (even in small doses) and NSAIDs as well as by anticoagulants.
- First aid involves pinching the nostrils together, not pressing on the nasal bridge.
- Anterior bleeds may be controlled by cautery or by an anterior nasal pack.
- Posterior bleeds may be controlled by an anterior nasal pack, or occasionally require both posterior and anterior nasal packs.
- Family practitioners should carry Merocel packs in their emergency bags.
- Be aware of adult patients with epistaxes associated with other nasal symptoms.

Consider referring

- Persisting epistaxis despite attempts to stop it.
- Patient actively bleeding requiring intravenous fluids and resuscitation.
- Recurrent epistaxes with no identifiable cause.
- Patient with epistaxes associated with other nasal symptoms.

The blocked nose

Nasal obstruction may be related to a mechanical or anatomical problem, or to a mucosal problem. In practice it is often a combination of both.

- If the problem is mechanical or anatomical, the blockage is usually unilateral and continuous. Causes include a deviated nasal septum, unilateral nasal polyp and nasal tumours (all discussed later in this section).

- If the problem is mucosal, the blockage tends to be intermittent and may go from side to side or be bilateral. The usual cause of a mucosal problem is rhinitis (discussed in the section on *The runny blocked nose*, page 95).

Normal nasal cycle: nasal airflow varies from one side to the other throughout the day and a nasal cycle of fluctuating nasal blockage may be demonstrated in almost everyone at rest. It results from variations in the amount of blood in the venous sinusoids in the nasal mucosa of the turbinates and septum, and is mediated by the autonomic nervous system.

History
Is the blockage continuous or does it fluctuate? If the blockage is continuous, it suggests that the problem is a structural one, i.e. it is there all the time. In adults this would commonly be related to a deviated nasal septum (usually unilateral obstruction) or to nasal polyps (usually bilateral). In children adenoidal hypertrophy would lead to persistent bilateral obstruction. If the problem fluctuates (especially from side to side) then it is likely to be related to a mucosal problem such as rhinitis.

Does it affect one or both sides? Persistent unilateral obstruction may be caused by a deviated nasal septum, unilateral polyp or a nasal tumour. Intermittent unilateral obstruction may be caused by rhinitis. Persistent bilateral obstruction suggests polyps in adults, enlarged adenoids in children.

Is the blockage associated with other symptoms? If associated with rhinorrhoea, sneezing bouts or itching, then the obstruction is more likely to be related to rhinitis. If associated with hyposmia/anosmia then nasal polyps are likely to be the underlying problem.

Examination

Examination of the external appearance of the nose may provide some clues to the cause of the obstruction.

■ An external deviation may be related to a corresponding deformity of the nasal septum.

■ Assessment of the airway and anterior rhinoscopy should allow differentiation between a deviated nasal septum, nasal polyps and rhinitis.

■ An inferior turbinate is sometimes mistaken for a polyp and the two can be differentiated using a nasal speculum and a probe: polyps are insensitive to touch and are mobile, whereas turbinates are tender and immobile.

Assessment in the ENT department

A flexible or rigid nasendoscope allows better visualization within the nose and assessment of the postnasal space. Occasionally even endoscopic examination does not provide a diagnosis, and in this situation a CT scan of the nose and paranasal sinuses may be useful.

Deviated nasal septum

A deviated nasal septum (Figure 3.4) is a relatively common finding and may be developmental or related to trauma. Unilateral nasal obstruction is the main complaint, but the obstruction may be bilateral if the deflected septum is s-shaped. Examination usually reveals not only the deviated septum but often compensatory hypertrophy of the inferior turbinate on the opposite side.

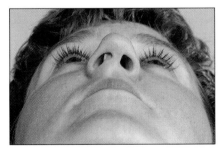

Treatment: an asymptomatic deviation obviously needs no treatment. If it is symptomatic, surgery is likely to be the only

Figure 3.4 *Deviated nasal septum. The caudal end of the nasal septum is displaced into the right nostril.*

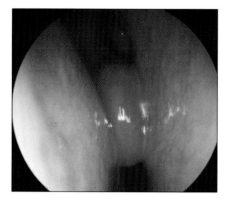

Figure 3.5 *Simple inflammatory nasal polyp.*

successful treatment. To avoid alterations to the shape of the growing nose, patients under 16 years old should not be referred for surgery.

The classical operation for correcting a deviation is the submucous resection (SMR), involving the removal of the deviated cartilage/bone. In septoplasty the cartilage excision is more conservative, so this operation may be preferred if it is considered necessary to maintain the supportive function of the septum.

Nasal polyps

These are 'bags' of oedematous mucosa, most commonly arising from the ethmoid sinuses and visible in the middle meatus, although when they are large they may fill the nose and appear at the external nares (Figure 3.5). They are usually multiple and bilateral and their pathogenesis is unclear. The cardinal symptom is progressive nasal obstruction and they eventually produce hyposmia/anosmia.

Examination and referral: examination is usually diagnostic, revealing structures similar to 'peeled grapes' within the nose, which are insensitive to touch and mobile (as opposed to inferior turbinates).

An ENT opinion should be sought at an early stage if the patient has a unilateral polyp, as it is possible for this to be a neoplastic polyp (Figure 3.6) as opposed to an inflammatory polyp. For the same reason, bleeding polyps should also be referred at an early stage. Patients whose polyps have failed to respond to medical treatment should be referred for consideration for surgery.

Medical treatment: if polyps are large and causing severe obstructive symptoms, then a short course of oral dexamethasone

- 8 mg per day for 4 days
- 4 mg per day for 4 days
- 2 mg per day for 4 days

can provide rapid reduction in polyp size and enable topical steroids to work. This should be followed by a 6–8 week course of betamethasone sodium 0.1% drops (Betnesol). It is important to instruct the patient to insert the drops in a correct head-down position (Figure 3.7) so that the medication reaches the middle meatal and ethmoidal areas. As the condition improves, a topical steroid spray such as beclomethasone diproprionate (Beconase) or fluticasone proprionate (Flixonase) can be substituted for the drops.

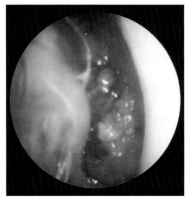

Figure 3.6 *A neoplastic nasal polyp.*

Surgical treatment involves removing the polyps in a conventional manner using a headlight, or endoscopically using rigid Hopkin's rods (endoscopes) to carry out endoscopic ethmoidectomy. Whatever

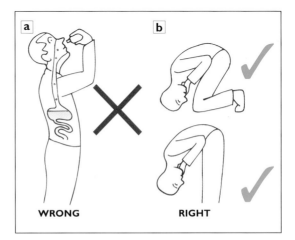

Figure 3.7 *Head-down position for the use of nose drops. (a) Incorrect position. (b) Correct head-down position.*

93

treatment is used, the polyps tend to recur eventually.

Nasal tumours

Urgent referral is indicated if a nasal tumour is suspected. They may present with:

- unilateral nasal obstruction
- unilateral epistaxis
- epiphora
- loosening of the teeth.

Key points

- Nasal obstruction may be related to a mechanical or anatomical problem, to a mucosal problem, or a combination of the two.
- A nasal cycle of fluctuating nasal blockage may be demonstrated in almost everyone at rest.
- A continuous blockage suggests a mechanical or anatomical problem, while a fluctuating one suggests a mucosal problem.
- An asymptomatic deviated nasal septum requires no treatment; surgery is likely to be the only successful treatment for one which is symptomatic.
- Nasal polyps should be differentiated from inferior turbinates.

Consider referring

- Symptomatic deviated nasal septum in patients over 16 years old.
- Nasal polyps where medical treatment has failed (for consideration of surgical removal).
- Unilateral or bleeding nasal polyps (to exclude nasal tumours).
- Any suspected nasal tumours.

The runny blocked nose

The runny blocked nose is usually caused by rhinitis, a very common problem that affects over 15% of the population in the UK. The term rhinitis implies an inflammatory response of the lining membrane of the nose, the aetiology of the response being variable. The patient presents with a runny nose which is often associated with intermittent nasal obstruction and other rhinitic symptoms (Table 3.1).

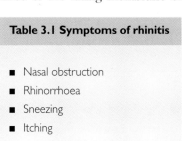

Table 3.1 Symptoms of rhinitis

- Nasal obstruction
- Rhinorrhoea
- Sneezing
- Itching

Classification of rhinitis

There is great confusion about the terminology used in classifying rhinitis. It would seem reasonable to consider three main groups: infective, allergic and intrinsic rhinitis.

Infective rhinitis: apart from acute viral rhinitis (including the common cold) this is a relatively unusual cause of rhinitis and is rarely a cause of chronic rhinitis.

Allergic rhinitis is an IgE-mediated hypersensitivity disease of the mucous membrane of the nasal airways characterized by:

- sneezing
- itching of the nose, eyes, throat, ears
- watery nasal discharge (may produce nocturnal cough)
- sensation of nasal obstruction (usually bilateral, but may alternate from side to side).

It occurs in atopic individuals and may be associated with allergic conjunctivitis and asthma. Allergic rhinitis may be either *seasonal* (e.g. hay fever) or *perennial* (in the UK, most commonly due to sensitivity to house dust mite). Seasonal allergic rhinitis can be caused by different

Table 3.2 Examples of allergens responsible for seasonal allergic rhinitis in the UK

- Spring — tree pollens (e.g. birch, hazel, ash)
- June/July — peak grass pollen counts
- Late summer — weed pollens (e.g. nettle, dock)
- Late summer/autumn — fungal spores

allergens at different times of the year (Table 3.2), and a patient allergic to more than one allergen may present with perennial symptoms.

Intrinsic rhinitis is a non-infective, non-allergic condition whose aetiology is obscure. It has been bedevilled by many names including perennial rhinitis and vasomotor rhinitis.

The main symptoms include:

- nasal congestion (usually bilateral but may alternate from side to side)
- rhinorrhoea
- postnasal discharge (posterior rhinorrhoea)
- hyposmia (poor sense of smell).

Sneezing and itching are less common and usually suggest an allergic rhinitis.

Diagnosis

The diagnosis (Figure 3.8) is largely dependent upon the history. The lack of unequivocal physical signs in this condition makes differentiation between the different types of rhinitis on the basis of examination difficult. The presence of seasonal variation, significant sneezing, nasal itching and a family history of atopy are highly suggestive of an allergic basis for the rhinitis.

Examination of the nose reveals an oedematous, congested nasal mucosa with increased (usually clear) nasal secretions. The mucosa

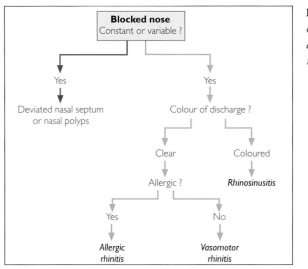

Figure 3.8 *Flow chart for diagnosis of a runny blocked nose.*

of the inferior turbinates is often so hypertrophied that it fills the anterior nares and touches the septum.

Treatment

The mainstay of treatment is medical, and the vast majority of patients can be treated in family practice without the need for referral.

Allergen avoidance should be attempted whenever it is practical (e.g. if a single allergen is recognized as the cause of an allergic rhinitis).

Medical treatment is similar for rhinitis of both allergic and non-allergic aetiology, and predominantly involves the use of topical steroids and antihistamines. To prevent any unrealistic expectations it is important to explain to the patient at the outset that treatment is designed to suppress symptoms rather than cure the condition.

Surgery to improve the nasal airway has only a limited role, and continuing medical treatment after any surgical intervention is usually essential to maintain any improvement in symptoms.

Allergen avoidance may be possible in perennial allergic rhinitis (e.g. when caused by feathers). In seasonal allergic rhinitis indoor exposure to pollen can be reduced by advising patients to keep doors and bedroom windows closed.

The major sources of house dust mite are mattresses, pillows and bed covers. Other sources include carpets and soft furnishings throughout the home. In order to reduce mite allergen levels the British Society of Allergy and Clinical Immunology recommends:

- bedding barrier intervention
- regular vacuuming of carpets and soft furnishings
- use of cork, vinyl or hardwood floors as alternatives to carpets.

Topical corticosteroids are extremely effective in controlling all nasal symptoms of allergic rhinitis in the majority of patients. They include beclomethasone (Beconase), budesonide (Rhinocort), flunisolide (Syntaris) and fluticasone (Flixonase). Fluticasone has the advantage of being effective once daily but is more expensive. Betamethasone nose drops (used in the head down and forward position) may also be effective.

Occasionally symptoms are so severe that a short course of oral steroids may be justified, e.g. in a teenager sitting important examinations.

Side-effects of topical corticosteroids are minimal. There is little evidence of a significant systemic steroid effect and local side-effects are not usually troublesome. Small epistaxes may occur but are much less common now that aqueous nasal sprays have become the preparation of choice (as opposed to propellant inhalers). There is no evidence that they cause atrophic rhinitis nor that they cause an increase in the incidence of bacterial or fungal infection in the nose or paranasal sinuses.

There are three common reasons for treatment failures.

- The medication has not been taken regularly: it is important to explain the prophylactic nature of the treatment to the patient.
- The patient has not persevered with the medication: compliance is often poor initially, and the necessity for a trial of at least 6 weeks should be explained.

- Faulty inhaler technique, caused by most patients thinking that the nasal airway runs vertically up the nose. They should be instructed to use the spray in the middle of a gentle inspiration, with the first spray directed along the floor of the nose parallel to the roof of the mouth, and the second directed towards the vault.

Antihistamines are particularly effective for the symptoms of sneezing, itching and watery rhinorrhoea, and also for the eye, palate and throat symptoms of allergic rhinitis. They have little effect on nasal congestion and blockage.

First-generation antihistamines have been largely superseded by the newer non-sedating forms, including:
- terfenadine, which is relatively inexpensive and effective (but in rare cases can cause dysrrhythmias in combination with other drugs, including erythromycin)
- astemizole, which is an effective alternative with a long half-life that can therefore be used once daily (it has rarely been associated with dysrhythmias)
- cetirizine (Zirtek), loratidine (Clarityn) and acrivastine (Semprex), which are all newer alternatives.

Antihistamines in topical form as nasal sprays (e.g. Azelastine, Rhinolast) offer no great advantage over oral preparations.

Topical vasoconstrictors: alpha-adrenoreceptor agonists (ephedrine, xylometazoline) are effective for nasal blockage but should be used for short periods of 2–3 weeks only. Longer courses may lead to problems with rhinitis medicamentosa, where patients need to use increasing amounts of the spray, which eventually loses its effect.

In the first 2 weeks of a course of topical steroids, severe nasal obstruction may prevent the effective use of the corticosteroid spray. It is often useful, therefore, to prescribe a topical vasoconstrictor for use 15–30 minutes before the steroid nasal spray is used.

Topical anticholinergics: ipratropium bromide (Rinatec) is often effective for watery rhinorrhoea.

Sodium cromoglycate: this mast cell-stabilising agent is sometimes an effective alternative to topical steroids. It is said to be particularly helpful in children.

Management of rhinitis in the ENT department

Referral may be required for patients with significant persisting symptoms despite adequate medical treatment.

Examination and diagnosis: the nose is examined using Hopkins' rigid rod telescopes (Figure 3.9). The endoscopic view provides additional information about the areas of the nose that are difficult to visualize with anterior rhinoscopy, and helps to exclude other possible problems such as nasal polyps or a posterior septal deviation.

A purulent nasal discharge associated with facial pain may suggest sinusitis and CT scanning would be used to investigate this.

In some ENT departments skin prick testing of common allergens (grass and tree pollen, house dust mite, dog hair and cat fur) will be performed. The value of these tests lies in providing supportive evidence for a diagnosis of allergic rhinitis.

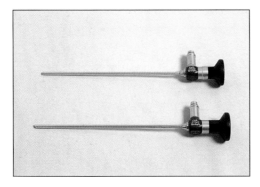

Figure 3.9 *The Hopkins' rod. These rigid telescopes have different viewing angles and those shown are 0 degree (straight ahead viewing) and 30 degrees. These are most commonly used for outpatient examination.*

Surgery: clearly surgical correction of any co-existent nasal problems will lessen the impact of the rhinitis itself. In the absence of such co-existing disease, surgery has only a limited role to play when intensive medical treatment has failed to relieve the patient's symptoms. Only a small minority of patients will need to be considered for surgical enlargement of the nasal airway by submucus diathermy and trimming of the inferior turbinates to reduce their mass.

Very rarely the problem of profuse rhinorrhoea may be reduced by interrupting the parasympathetic nerve supply to the nose (vidian neurectomy), although its value is subject to debate.

Key points

- Rhinitis is a very common problem, affecting over 15% of the population in the UK.
- Allergic rhinitis may be perennial (usually related to house dust mite) or seasonal (usually related to pollen).
- Intrinsic rhinitis is a non-infective, non-allergic condition whose aetiology is obscure.
- Diagnosis is largely dependent on the history.
- The mainstay of treatment of allergic and intrinsic rhinitis is medical and is often designed to suppress symptoms rather than cure the condition.
- Medical treatment predominantly involves the use of topical corticosteroids and antihistamines.
- Surgery has only a limited role in rhinitis.
- In family practice, a systematic approach should be effective in diagnosing and treating the majority of patients with rhinitis.

Consider referring

- Patients with persisting symptoms and treatment failures.
- If co-existing problems such as a deviated nasal septum or nasal polyps are suspected.
- If chronic sinusitis is suspected.
- Where skin prick testing may be helpful.

Facial pain

The patient with facial pain can present a diagnostic challenge, and in a large proportion of cases there will be no identifiable pathology.

Facial pain may be related to some localized pathology or referred from some other area of the head and neck. Painful stimuli affecting facial structures are transmitted via afferents in the fifth cranial nerve to the spinal tract in the brain stem. Pain afferents also run in cranial nerves VII, IX and X. When trying to identify the cause of the pain it is essential to take a detailed history and to look at the site of the pain to identify any local disease. If no local cause is detected, then the remainder of the head and neck must be examined to exclude the causes of referred pain (Figure 3.10).

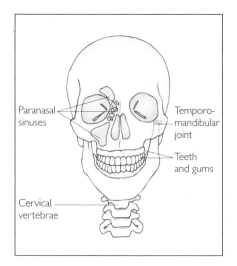

Paranasal sinuses

Temporo-mandibular joint

Teeth and gums

Cervical vertebrae

Figure 3.10 *Common sites of pathology causing referred facial/head and neck pain.*

Working classification of the causes of facial pain

These causes primarily result in local pain but can also present as pain elsewhere in the head and neck.

Rhinological pain
- Sinusitis
- Chronic rhinosinusitis
- Malignant rhinologic disease

Dental pain
- Local dental disease
- Temporomandibular joint dysfunction

Vascular pain
- Migraine
- Cluster headaches
- Temporal arteritis

Neuralgias
- Trigeminal neuralgia
- Glossopharyngeal neuralgia
- Post-herpetic neuralgia

Central pain

Ophthalmic pain

Miscellaneous facial pain
- Tension headache
- Atypical facial pain

Rhinological pain

Sinusitis: sinus pain is usually reasonably well localized — the exception being pain related to the sphenoid sinus.

Acute sinusitis of the *maxillary or ethmoid sinuses* usually produces local discomfort over the cheeks and nasal bridge, and most commonly follows a cold. The pain is often exacerbated by bending down or by moving the eyes from side to side, and the maxillary teeth often ache. Examination often shows maxillary or frontal sinus tenderness, but rarely swelling of the overlying soft tissues unless there is complicating osteomyelitis. Mucopus may be visible in the nose, particularly in the middle meatus under the middle turbinate. Occasionally the discharge may be blood-stained.

Eye movements and visual acuity should be checked for possible orbital complications.

Plain sinus X-rays have little place in the management of sinusitis in family practice: a CT scan is the only radiological investigation that will show sufficient detail.

Treatment in family practice with broad spectrum antibiotics in combination with vasoconstricting drops or inhalations is usually successful.

Chronic rhinosinusitis may be associated with few symptoms other than nasal congestion and rhinorrhoea (which may be purulent, and affect both anterior and posterior nares), but is sometimes the cause of long-standing facial pain.

Referral for CT scanning will identify the more subtle changes characteristic of this condition. A CT scan will also identify patients with diseased ethmoidal sinuses who may benefit from ethmoidectomy by functional endoscopic sinus surgery (FESS).

Treatment in family practice with a 2–3 week course of antibiotics and 2–3 months of a topical steroid may settle symptoms, but recurrent episodes or persistent symptoms necessitate referral.

Malignant rhinologic disease: maxillary and nasopharyngeal malignancy are rare causes of facial pain.

Dental pain

Local dental disease may be associated with pain and hypersensitivity to hot or cold stimuli. Dental pulp problems tend to produce poorly localized pain, whereas dentino-enamel defects initially produce a sharp, well-localized pain that is often followed by a dull ache.

Temporomandibular joint dysfunction is usually unilateral (in 90% of cases) and usually occurs in young adults with a history of bruxism, clenching, recent dental work or poor dental occlusion. Pain is caused by pterygoid muscle spasm and presents as a deep dull ache that may masquerade as toothache or earache. Examination shows tenderness over the joint and the pain is exacerbated by opening the mouth or chewing.

Treatment in family practice with anti-inflammatory analgesics may help, and most patients respond when aggravating factors are corrected. Referral to the oral surgery department for occlusal devices may be necessary if simple measures fail.

Vascular pain

Migraine may present with hemifacial pain in the frontal area as well as in the temporal or parietal regions. A positive family history, the presence of prodromal symptoms, and associated nausea, visual disturbance and other neurological symptoms will point towards the diagnosis.

Cluster headaches usually present with severe unilateral stabbing or burning pain which may be frontal, temporal, ocular, over the cheek or even in the maxillary teeth. Nausea is usually absent but frequently there is rhinorrhoea, conjunctival injection and lacrimation with unilateral nasal obstruction.

Treatment with a combination of a NSAID and amitriptyline at night is often helpful.

Temporal arteritis causes pain in the temporal region, and classically the temporal artery is tender and thickened. The erythrocyte sedimentation rate (ESR) and C-reactive protein (CRP) are markedly raised, and if the diagnosis is uncertain then urgent biopsy of the artery is indicated.

Treatment is with oral steroids which should not be withheld whilst waiting for the test results.

Neuralgias

Trigeminal neuralgia: patients complain of paroxysms of agonising lancinating pain induced by a specific trigger point. It can often be treated successfully with carbamazepine.

Glossopharyngeal neuralgia is uncommon. Pain is felt in the tonsillar region and in the ipsilateral ear, and may be precipitated by swallowing or talking.

Post-herpetic neuralgia is more common in the elderly. If it persists for more than a year it is unlikely to resolve completely.

Central pain

Stretching of the arteries supplying the proximal cranial nerves and the dura induces a headache but can also cause facial pain. Space-occupying lesions can induce facial pain by irritation of the trigeminal nerve along its intracerebral course.

Ophthalmic pain

Inflammatory and infective eye diseases cause ophthalmic pain and characteristic eye changes. Glaucoma can cause severe orbital and peri-orbital pain. Pain is also a feature of peri-orbital cellulitis which may present with lid-swelling and erythema if it is preseptal, and with chemosis, proptosis and reduced mobility if it arises posterior to the septum.

Miscellaneous facial pain

Tension headache is one of the commonest causes of pain over the forehead, eyes or temples. It is typically described as a feeling of tightness or pressure often distributed in a band around the head. The family practitioner is in the ideal position to explore the contributing stresses in the patient's life.

Atypical facial pain is a diagnosis made only when organic causes have been excluded. The pain is typically deep and ill-defined, may change location, is not usually confined to any one nerve distribution, and has no precipitating or relieving factors. Treatment with a tricyclic antidepressant often helps the pain.

Key points

- The pain may be related to some localized pathology or may be referred.
- In a large proportion of individuals there will be no identifiable pathology.

Consider referring

- When a definitive diagnosis cannot be made and the pain persists.
- When a serious underlying cause for the pain is suspected.
- Chronic rhinosinusitis causing recurrent or persistent symptoms.
- Where the presumed diagnosis necessitates referral for a dental, oral surgical, neurological or ophthalmic opinion.

Chapter 4

The mouth and throat

Common lesions of the oral cavity

Patients often present to their family practitioners with oral symptoms and most lesions in the mouth will be visible or palpable to both the patient and clinician.

Symptoms of oral disease

Pain: dental disease is the commonest cause of pain in the mouth. As well as causing pain, periodontal disease can produce halitosis because of an accumulation of decaying food debris. Aphthous ulcers are often a cause of moderately severe pain, whereas early malignancy is not painful.

Oral masses: any complaint of a lump requires palpation of the site, even if a lesion is not visible. If the mass is palpable it will probably require biopsy to provide a histological diagnosis.

Ulceration: aphthous ulcers are the commonest cause of oral ulcers seen in family practice and they should heal in 2 weeks. Any ulcer that persists for 3 weeks should be considered malignant until proven otherwise and warrants urgent referral.

Haemorrhage is frequently due to gum disease secondary to dental caries, but may be related to malignancy. Any patient complaining of recurrently tasting or finding blood in the mouth requires careful examination of the nose and oral cavity. If no cause of the bleeding is found then referral for endoscopic examination of the nose, postnasal space and larynx is indicated.

Halitosis: poor dental hygiene is the main cause. Advanced oral/oropharyngeal malignant disease can be associated with an offensive smell.

Burning mouth: family practitioners will be familiar with patients complaining of a burning mouth ('burning mouth syndrome'). The mouth looks normal on examination, and the symptom is often eased by drinking water or by eating. There may be a psychological element, and some reports have suggested deficiency of iron, or of folic acid, vitamin B^{12} or other B vitamins.

Ageusia: inability to taste is rarely associated with oral disease alone. More commonly it presents in patients with nasal pathology where the sense of smell (which is responsible for most of the qualitative sense of taste) has been affected.

Causes of ulceration in the oral cavity

- Recurrent aphthous stomatitis
- Infections
- Trauma (e.g. poorly-fitting dentures)
- Agranulocytosis
- Neutropenia
- Behçet's disease
- Erythema multiforme/Stevens–Johnson syndrome

Recurrent aphthous stomatitis

This is the commonest cause of ulcers of the oral cavity, affecting up to 20% of the population, in particular students and members of upper socio-economic groups. Aphthous ulcers are unusual after the age of 60, so should be treated with suspicion if they present in elderly patients.

Characteristics: aphthous ulcers:

- are associated with severe pain
- are typically round or oval in shape, 1–2 mm in diameter, with a whitish base and surrounding erythematous halo but no surrounding hyperkeratosis or induration
- affect buccal mucosa or tongue (an ulcer on the palate is not aphthous)
- usually present 1–5 at a time
- heal within 2 weeks
- may be associated with deficiencies of iron, folate or B^{12} (involved in epithelial formation)
- may be associated with malabsorption states (e.g. Crohn's disease, coeliac disease)
- may be related to food sensitivity (patch-testing and avoidance may help).

Investigations to exclude possible causes should include:

- full blood count and iron studies
- red cell folate and serum B^{12}
- endomysial antibodies (recurrent aphthous stomatitis may be the only clinical manifestation of coeliac disease).

Treatment is difficult and often not needed, but the following may be worth trying:

- frequent mouthwashes using saline or thymol and glycerin
- antiseptic mouthwashes (e.g. 0.2% chlorhexidine gluconate or 1% povidone-iodine)
- topical anaesthetic spray (e.g. benzydamine 0.15%)

- Adcortyl in Orabase (it is important to instruct the patient to apply the ointment with a wet finger to dry mucosa, as it only sticks to a dry mouth)
- topical steroid in the form of hydrocortisone lozenges 2.5 mg qds, or a mouthwash of triamcinolone acetonide 0.1% suspension, or a beclomethasone inhaler sprayed into the mouth.

Infections which can cause oral ulceration

HIV can cause ulcers identical to major aphthous ulcers.

Coxsackie virus infections: ulcers particularly affect the soft palate and oropharynx. In hand-foot-and-mouth disease they are associated with a vesicular eruption on the palms and soles, and sometimes the trunk.

Primary herpes stomatitis presents in children with widespread oral ulceration. It is usually so painful that the child is reluctant to drink.

Other infections: tuberculosis, syphilis and chronic fungal infections should be considered in atypical oral ulceration.

Mouth cancer

The incidence of oral and oropharyngeal cancer (Figure 4.1) in this country is rising, particularly in younger patients. It is important to remember that:

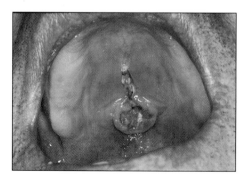

Figure 4.1 *Squamous cell carcinoma involving hard palate.*

- 70% of cases occur in heavy smokers and alcohol abusers
- any ulcer, red or white patch, or area of induration that persists longer than 3 weeks needs urgent referral
- malignancies are often found on the side of the tongue and/or on the floor of the mouth and it is vital that these sites are examined as a matter of routine
- fixation to underlying structures may cause limitation of tongue movement
- mortality can be reduced by early referral
- early cancer is not painful and often has a non-specific appearance.

Other lesions in the oral cavity

White lesions: the common lesions are:

- lichen planus, which produces a lacy white pattern on the buccal mucosa
- candidiasis (Figure 4.2), where the white patches can be wiped off (unlike those of lichen planus)
- leucoplakia (Figure 4.3), a white patch stuck to the tongue or oral mucosa which can be pre-malignant and requires biopsy.

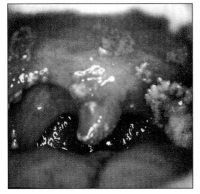

Figure 4.2 *Oral candidiasis.*

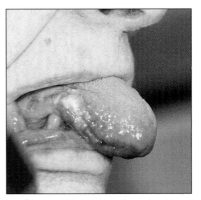

Figure 4.3 *Leucoplakia of the lateral border of the tongue.*

113

Red lesions include:

- geographical tongue, presenting as numerous red patches due to loss of papillae, with an outline that often changes, and requiring no treatment (although some cases respond to zinc sulphate mouthwash)
- median rhomboid glossitis, presenting as a red area just anterior to the circumvallate papillae in the midline and requiring no treatment.

Miscellaneous lesions include retention cysts, torus palatinus and black hairy tongue.

- Retention cysts can occur anywhere due to duct blockage of minor salivary glands. They can reach large sizes, especially if located in the floor of the mouth where the term 'ranula' (named after the bulging vocal pouch of a frog's throat) is applied (Figure 4.4).
- Torus palatinus is a bony exostosis in the midline of the hard palate. It may need removal if affecting the fitting of a denture. The rarer minor salivary gland tumours which occur at this site are often malignant, and are fairly firm but not bony hard.

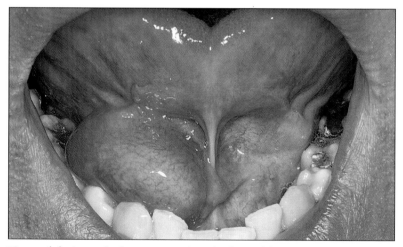

Figure 4.4 *A ranula (retention cyst) in the floor of the mouth.*

- Black hairy tongue presents most often in smokers. Treatment involves daily application of a toothbrush to the tongue, and anti-smoking advice. It may be caused by *Aspergillus niger* (e.g. after antibiotics).

Key points

- Any complaint of a lump in the oral cavity (whether visible or not) requires palpation of the site.
- Any oral ulcer or non-ulcerating mass that persists longer than 3 weeks needs urgent referral for biopsy.
- Beware oral ulcers in patients over 60 years of age.
- To exclude malignancy always examine the underneath of the tongue and ask the patient to deviate the extended tongue sideways.
- Early oral cancer is not painful.
- Patients with recurrent aphthous stomatitis should have their haematinics and endomysial antibodies checked.

Consider referring

- Any ulcer, red or white patch, area of induration, or mass that persists longer than 3 weeks.
- Any patient with white lesions in the oral cavity where a diagnosis of candidiasis or lichen planus cannot be made.
- Recurrent blood in the mouth where no cause is found.

Sore throat

Acute sore throat: causes

Acute sore throat is one of the commonest conditions seen in family practice and is usually (in about 70% of cases) due to a viral infection. The most common bacterial cause is the group A beta-haemolytic streptococcus *(Streptococcus pyogenes)*, which can be isolated from up to 30% of patients presenting with a sore throat, and from as many as 50% of children aged 4–13 years. Other causes of an exudative tonsillitis include infectious mononucleosis and (in rare cases) diphtheria.

It is notoriously difficult to distinguish between viral and bacterial sore throats on clinical grounds alone, but the following characteristics may support (although they do not prove) the diagnosis.

Acute viral sore throat is usually part of a viral upper respiratory tract infection with a variety of other coryzal symptoms including a runny nose, sneezing, hoarseness, a dry cough and dullness of hearing. There is often a generalized redness of the pharynx, tonsils and soft palate, and there may also be a petechial rash on the soft palate. Viral sore throats are more common in winter, and usually settle in about 3 days.

Acute streptococcal tonsillitis

has the following characteristics:
- pain of sudden onset
- dysphagia
- significant systemic symptoms such as fever and headache
- markedly red and congested oropharynx, and often pharyngeal or tonsillar exudate (Figure 4.5)
- enlarged tender cervical lymph nodes

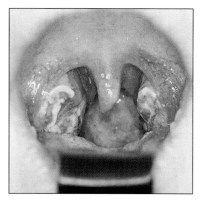

Figure 4.5 *Acute follicular tonsillitis with marked tonsillar exudate.*

- typical 'scarlet fever' rash
- referred otalgia is common
- halitosis.

The presence of a cough or of other coryzal symptoms decreases the probability of a streptococcal infection.

Infectious mononucleosis is commonly seen in teenagers, and characteristically the patient:

- has membranous exudate over the tonsils
- is systemically unwell
- has generalized lymphadenopathy and splenomegaly
- has atypical lymphocytes in the peripheral blood film, and positive monospot or Paul-Bunnell tests some days or even weeks after the onset
- may have abnormal liver function tests.

The possibility of infectious mononucleosis should not prevent penicillin being prescribed, but is a good reason to avoid amoxycillin, which can cause a very troublesome rash.

Diphtheria: although this is extremely rare in the UK, it may present in patients returning from countries where epidemics may be occurring.

Acute sore throat: investigations

Throat swabs: it is clearly not practical to take a throat swab from every patient presenting with a sore throat and the following arguments against routine swabbing can be put forward.

- If the family practitioner waits (usually 48 hours) for the result before prescribing treatment then it may be too late for antibiotics to have any benefit.
- Routine throat swabs would cost the NHS an additional £40–45 million a year.
- 5% of the population are healthy streptococcal carriers who are as likely as anyone else to develop a viral sore throat.

- Taking a throat swab may be unpleasant for patients (especially children) and this may make taking an adequate swab difficult.

However, throat swabs can be an important investigation in:
- patients with persisting or recurrent sore throats
- patients who are HIV positive or who are otherwise immunocompromised.

Anti-streptolysin O (ASO) titre rises too late to influence the immediate management of sore throat but can confirm recent streptococcal infection if the patient remains unwell.

C-reactive protein (CRP) increases rapidly and to higher levels with bacterial infections than with viral infections, but has little practical use at present in family practice.

Rapid antigen tests for streptococci are expensive, and cannot be prescribed in the UK. Their sensitivity and specificity has been questioned in family practice studies in Britain.

Acute sore throat: treatment

Self-care by patients: most sore throats will be self-limiting and management will be aimed at encouraging patients in self-care using paracetamol, saline gargles, and honey and lemon mixtures.

Antibiotics: the decision whether or not to prescribe antibiotics is based on clinical criteria, and on the probability that the patient has a streptococcal infection. As this is difficult to assess on clinical grounds alone, it is inevitable that some patients will be prescribed antibiotics unnecessarily while other patients with a streptococcal infection will not be given them.

Some family practitioners question the value and cost-effectiveness of treating patients with streptococcal sore throat with antibiotics. There is some, but not overwhelming, evidence that treating such patients with antibiotics does curtail the duration of symptoms. The family practitioner should attempt to discuss these issues with the patient (or the parents if the patient is a child) in an attempt to reduce antibiotic prescribing in patients suffering from sore throats.

Penicillin is the antibiotic of choice, with erythromycin as the alternative for patients allergic to penicillin. The standard advice is that a 10-day course is necessary completely to eradicate *S. pyogenes*, but in practice few patients will comply with this. Most patients will be prescribed a 5- or 7-day course, and it is reasonable to reserve longer courses for persisting or recurrent cases.

Amoxycillin should not be used because of the risk of causing a troublesome rash in glandular fever.

Complications of tonsillitis

Quinsy (peritonsillar abscess) (Figure 4.6) is almost always unilateral and results from spread of infection from the tonsil into the space between the tonsil and the adjacent constrictor muscle. Clinically the sore throat becomes unilateral, and this is associated with increasing dysphagia and trismus. The most obvious clinical sign is marked unilateral tonsillar inflammation causing deviation of the base of the uvula to the opposite side. As the abscess increases in size it involves the soft palate above the tonsillar fossa, and the parapharyngeal space infection can be seen as a marked swelling in the neck.

An early quinsy may be treated with 6-hourly intramuscular benzyl penicillin initially, changing to oral penicillin after 2–3 doses. It is also wise to add oral metronidazole.

Fully-developed quinsy requires hospital admission for intravenous antibiotics. If there is evidence of a collection of pus, then this should be drained under local anaesthetic using a wide bore needle and syringe.

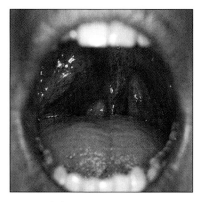

Figure 4.6 *A right-sided quinsy.*

Acute rheumatic fever and **acute glomerulonephritis** complicating streptococcal tonsillitis are now extremely rare in the UK. Their incidence declined well before antibiotics were introduced, and concern about patients developing these illnesses is therefore *not* a valid reason for prescribing antibiotics for patients with sore throats.

Tonsillectomy

The indications for surgery remain controversial. The family practitioner is in the ideal position to assess the severity and frequency of attacks of tonsillitis in any individual patient, and it is essential that the referral letter includes these details. The specialist's decision whether or not to operate depends largely on the history provided by the patient's family practitioner, and this has led some ENT departments to allow family practitioners direct access to tonsillectomy waiting lists.

Tonsillectomy: indications and contraindications

Indications for tonsillectomy

- Recurrent tonsillitis: usually 3–6 bouts per year for 2 years consecutively, although the severity of the attacks may mean that surgery is sometimes indicated at an earlier date. No one *has* to undergo tonsillectomy for this indication — it is a *relative* rather than an *absolute* indication. There is often spontaneous improvement as a child approaches the age of 10 years.
- Sleep apnoea secondary to adenotonsillar hypertrophy (large tonsils without apnoea are *not* an indication for surgery).
- Single quinsy with an associated history of recurrent tonsillitis, or more than one quinsy.
- Unilateral tonsillar enlargement or abnormality (to exclude neoplasia). Many patients have tonsils of asymmetrical size, and it is only when this is particularly marked and the tonsil

abnormal in appearance that referral is necessary.

Contraindications to tonsillectomy

- Bleeding disorders.
- Tonsillectomy is usually postponed if the patient has had tonsillitis within 2 weeks of admission for surgery, because of the increased risk of a secondary haemorrhage. Prophylactic penicillin may be prescribed for patients who have very frequent episodes of tonsillitis, to cover them for the 3 weeks before surgery.

Postoperative care: the policy in most ENT departments in the UK is to discharge patients on the first postoperative day. The most important advice to be given to the patient in the postoperative period is to take regular analgesia and to continue eating and drinking if at all possible.

It is usually only during the first postoperative week that the pain reaches its peak. Many patients (27% of patients undergoing tonsillectomy in one study) will present to their family practitioners at this stage with a history of becoming worse (rather than better) since their discharge from hospital. In addition they may have developed referred otalgia. On examination the oropharynx looks inflamed with a white 'healing' membrane over the site of the tonsils on each side (Figure 4.7), and it is easy for this to be mistaken for infection. Although antibiotics may have a part to play under some circumstances, it is more likely that increasing the strength of the patient's analgesics and promoting any measures that

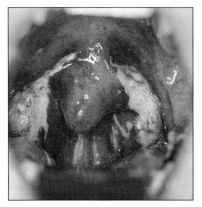

Figure 4.7 *Normal post-tonsillectomy appearance of the fauces.*

121

help oral hygiene will be the most useful treatment.

Postoperative bleeding usually occurs either within the first 24 hours during the patient's stay in hospital (primary or reactionary haemorrhage), or 5–10 days postoperatively (secondary haemorrhage). A history of secondary haemorrhage is obviously an absolute indication for urgent referral back to the ENT department.

Adenoidectomy
Large adenoids can cause nasal obstruction resulting in mouth breathing. As the Eustachian tubes open into the nasopharynx, large adenoids may play a part in the pathogenesis of recurrent acute otitis media and glue ear.

Indications for adenoidectomy
- Chronic nasal obstruction secondary to adenoidal hypertrophy. If there is also anterior nasal obstruction secondary to rhinitis, then adenoidectomy may not improve the breathing.
- Certain cases of glue ear and recurrent acute otitis media.
- Sleep apnoea (in conjunction with tonsillectomy).

Chronic sore throat
It can be difficult for family practitioners to decide whether or not patients are likely to have significant underlying pathology to account for their symptoms, especially as examination of the oral cavity and oropharynx will often be entirely normal. In many cases no obvious cause can be found even when the hypopharynx and larynx are examined in the ENT department.

Chronic pharyngitis is the commonest cause of a chronic sore throat in adults. This inflammation is usually multifactorial and non-infective. Smoke and alcohol are particularly irritant to the pharyngeal mucosa and are often aetiological factors. Oesophageal reflux is also sometimes associated with pharyngitis and treatment with a proton pump inhibitor will often cure both.

Chronically infected tonsils may cause a chronic sore throat but the place for tonsillectomy in this situation is much less clear-cut than in recurrent acute tonsillitis.

Referral: patients with persisting symptoms will need referral, especially if there are associated symptoms such as hoarseness, dysphagia, foreign body sensation or unilateral otalgia. The ENT specialist will be able to examine the larynx and hypopharynx with a mirror or flexible nasolaryngoscope. Further investigations may involve a barium swallow to assess the upper oesophagus, and a CT or MRI scan if appropriate.

Key points

- Most acute sore throats are viral in origin.
- The majority of patients with sore throats do not require antibiotics.
- Routine throat swabs are not helpful.
- Quinsy requires treatment with parenteral antibiotics and drainage of any pus collection.
- Post-tonsillectomy, it is normal to see a white membrane over the site of the tonsils and this is not a sign of infection.
- Chronic pharyngitis is the commonest cause of a chronic sore throat.

Consider referring

- Patients who would benefit from adenotonsillectomy.
- Secondary haemorrhage following tonsillectomy.
- Any patient with a chronic sore throat who also has hoarseness, dysphagia, foreign body sensation or unilateral otalgia.

Snoring and sleep apnoea

'Laugh and the world laughs with you, snore and you sleep alone'
(Anon.)
Most adults snore occasionally, but there are those who snore on a regular basis for whom the social consequences can be extremely distressing. Indeed, the main problem of snoring is a social one, with the consultation often being prompted by the patient's partner. (It is worth remembering in these circumstances that sometimes complaining of a partner's snoring provides an excuse for no longer sharing a bed, and that the actual amount of snoring involved may be trivial.) Family practitioners are likely to see an increasing number of patients presenting with this complaint as public awareness and expectation of a 'cure' continue to rise, and more is written in the popular press on the treatment options.

Among the group of patients who snore regularly are a few who develop obstructive sleep apnoea (OSA) syndrome: this diagnosis needs to be considered in all those who habitually snore (Table 4.1).

Mechanism
During sleep the pharyngeal airway narrows (Figure 4.8) due to a reduction in dilator muscle tone. If this reduction in tone is marked, snoring results from the vibration of pharyngeal structures such as the uvula and soft palate, tongue base and pharyngeal walls.

Further narrowing produces louder snoring and laboured inspiration, and eventually complete obstruction with apnoeic spells. The brain senses the increased inspiratory effort after 10–15 seconds and the individual

Table 4.1 Indicators of sleep apnoea

- Daytime sleepiness
- Regularly waking unrefreshed
- Partner describes typical apnoeic episodes
- Men with collar size 17^1/2 or larger

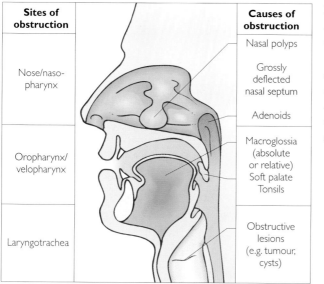

Sites of obstruction	Causes of obstruction
Nose/naso-pharynx	Nasal polyps Grossly deflected nasal septum Adenoids
Oropharynx/velopharynx	Macroglossia (absolute or relative) Soft palate Tonsils
Laryngotrachea	Obstructive lesions (e.g. tumour, cysts)

Figure 4.8
Potential sites and causes of narrowing that may result in snoring and obstructive sleep apnoea.

partially arouses. There may be hundreds of such arousals in one night causing severe sleep disturbance and thus greatly impaired daytime performance at work, at home and when driving. During the apnoeic spells there is significant hypoxia which can result in right heart strain.

Causes of snoring

Snoring becomes more common with increasing age, mainly because of the increased laxity of soft tissue. Approximately 25% of men and 15% of women snore habitually, and this frequency doubles in those who are overweight or over 65 years of age. Other causes include:

- evening alcohol
- obesity
- smoking
- menopause
- poor nasal airway (e.g. deviated septum, rhinitis, polyps)
- hypothyroidism
- receding lower jaw.

125

Management of snoring

Initial treatment should include lifestyle advice:

- weight reduction
- stopping smoking
- stopping evening alcohol
- sleeping with the head of the bed elevated to reduce nasal congestion.

Where appropriate:

- the nasal airway may be improved by using topical corticosteroids
- the patient's thyroid function should be checked
- HRT should be considered.

Referral for surgery: if simple measures fail then referral may be appropriate as some patients may consider surgery.

If significant nasal obstruction exists then surgery aimed at improving this may be enough. However, in many patients surgery to the palate and lateral pharyngeal walls may be required to help their snoring. In uvulopalatopharyngoplasty (UPPP) redundant tissues in the soft palate and lateral pharyngeal walls are trimmed away, including the tonsils if present (Figure 4.9). UPPP is successful in helping to reduce the volume of snoring in 90% of patients. In many surgical units this surgery would not be performed without the patient first being fully assessed in a sleep laboratory to confirm snoring and to exclude the possibility of obstructive sleep apnoea (this type of surgery is not appropriate treatment for OSA).

Obstructive sleep apnoea (OSA)

Management: as with simple snoring, loss of weight and reduction in alcohol intake will help.

Nasal continuous positive airway pressure (CPAP) consists of a small mask fitting over the nose and mouth connected to a pump that ensures that the pressure in the upper airway remains positive, therefore avoiding obstruction.

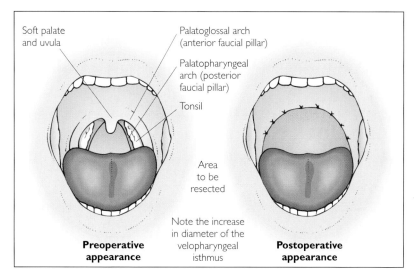

Soft palate and uvula
Palatoglossal arch (anterior faucial pillar)
Palatopharyngeal arch (posterior faucial pillar)
Tonsil
Area to be resected
Note the increase in diameter of the velopharyngeal isthmus
Preoperative appearance
Postoperative appearance

Figure 4.9 *The appearance of the oropharynx before and after uvulopalatopharyngoplasty (UPPP).*

OSA in children: sleep apnoea with snoring is common in children of 2–6 years of age when they have upper respiratory infections that cause the tonsils to enlarge.

In some children the adenoids and tonsils are permanently enlarged and cause the problem every night. This can result in daytime sleepiness, bad behaviour, hyperactivity and a poor attention span.

With a classical history and the finding of large, obstructing tonsils on examination, referral to the ENT department is indicated. Adenotonsillectomy is curative. If there is doubt about the diagnosis then referral for sleep studies is advisable.

Key points

■ Snoring is more common in those who are overweight, drink excessive alcohol or smoke.

■ If troublesome snoring persists after weight loss and reduced alcohol intake, surgery may be helpful.

■ OSA may cause daytime sleepiness and secondary cardiac complications.

■ OSA in adults is usually treated with nasal CPAP.

■ OSA in children is usually cured by adenotonsillectomy.

Consider referring

■ Patients where weight loss and reduced alcohol intake have not helped reduce the snoring and who wish to consider UPPP.

■ Patients with nasal obstruction (to consider nasal surgery).

■ Adults with significant OSA to a sleep clinic (for possible nasal CPAP).

■ Children with significant OSA (for adenotonsillectomy).

Dysphagia

Assessment and diagnosis

It is important to establish the precise symptoms in patients who present with dysphagia. Such patients fall into two groups:

■ those complaining of feelings of a lump in the throat (often localized at the suprasternal notch) not associated with true dysphagia, e.g. patients with globus pharyngeus

■ those complaining of true dysphagia, i.e. difficulty swallowing.

Clearly true dysphagia would suggest a more sinister cause and necessitate urgent referral. However, because of the relative size of the mouth and pharynx, lesions in these areas (as opposed to lesions of the oesophagus) rarely cause total obstruction to the passage of food, and instead more frequently give rise to a foreign body sensation in the throat. For this reason, patients complaining of such sensations will also need urgent investigation if the symptoms persist for more than about 4 weeks. In particular, any patient who has a foreign body sensation or dysphagia in combination with hoarseness, unilateral otalgia or a neck mass warrants urgent referral (Figure 4.10).

Because total obstruction to the passage of food is rare in pharyngeal malignant disease it is less commonly associated with significant weight loss than is an oesophageal pathology.

Examination and referral: examination may make the diagnosis clear in diseases of the oral cavity and oropharynx. If this examination is normal and the neck is clear, it is reasonable to arrange for an urgent barium swallow for patients complaining of a

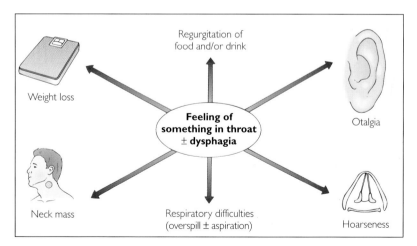

Figure 4.10 *Symptoms requiring full investigation if associated with foreign body sensation/dysphagia.*

lump in the throat/foreign body sensation. If this proves normal and the symptoms resolve then no further investigation is needed.

If symptoms persist, even in the presence of a normal barium swallow, then referral for further assessment of the larynx and hypopharynx will be required.

Assessment in the ENT department: the upper aerodigestive tract will be assessed by mirror examination or flexible nasolaryngoscopy. If there is any doubt following this outpatient assessment, the patient may be admitted for rigid endoscopy under general anaesthesia.

Causes of dysphagia

Acute dysphagia
- Infections such as pharyngitis and tonsillitis
- May be related to an ingested foreign body

Chronic dysphagia
- Neuromuscular disorders
- Intrinsic lesions
  - Neoplasia
  - Pharyngeal pouch
  - Globus pharyngeus

Neuromuscular disorders

Many neurological disorders can affect swallowing: the following are those most commonly seen in family practice.
- In the elderly neuromuscular dysfunction in the pharynx and upper oesophagus is often the cause and can be demonstrated on barium swallow with video.
- Cerebrovascular accident. If the dysphagia is severe and in danger

of causing pulmonary aspiration then a feeding gastrostomy may be necessary.

■ Motor neurone disease. There are usually other manifestations of the disease to suggest the diagnosis. The management of the dysphagia may again involve a feeding gastrostomy and occasionally cricopharyngeal myotomy.

Intrinsic lesions

Neoplasia of the pharynx and oesophagus may cause dysphagia alone, but will often produce other symptoms such as hoarseness or referred otalgia. It is notoriously difficult for patients to localize the site of dysphagia, often pointing to, for example, the mid-sternum when the lesion is in the pharynx.

Pharyngeal pouch is a hernia of the pharyngeal mucosa through a potential weakness in the pharyngeal muscle layers. Food debris collects in the pouch and the patient may complain of the regurgitation of food and chronic cough (related to overspill of secretions into the larynx) as well as dysphagia. A barium swallow is diagnostic (Figure 4.11).

Small pouches causing minimal symptoms do not require treatment. Pouches producing significant symptoms may be treated surgically either via an external approach or endoscopically.

Globus pharyngeus is an extremely common condition. The patient has a feeling of a lump in the throat, often localized to the level of the

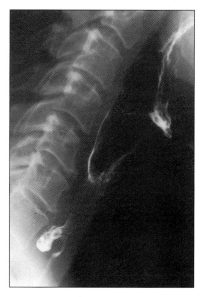

Figure 4.11 *Barium swallow demonstrating a small pharyngeal pouch.*

131

suprasternal notch. True dysphagia is not present — indeed the 'lump' often disappears during eating and is more pronounced when swallowing saliva.

The underlying pathology is not understood but in some cases it is possible that oesophageal reflux may induce cricopharyngeal spasm (hence some advocate a trial of anti-reflux therapy).

Often the reassurance of a normal barium swallow and meal is enough to help the patient, but clearly if symptoms persist referral for further investigation is indicated.

Key points

- Significant lesions in the pharynx often give rise to a foreign body sensation in the throat without initially causing true dysphagia.
- Significant weight loss is rare in pharyngeal malignant disease until it is reasonably advanced.
- In patients with foreign body sensation without true dysphagia it is reasonable to arrange an urgent barium swallow if symptoms persist for more than 4 weeks and no local cause can be found on examination.
- If symptoms persist even in the presence of a normal barium swallow then urgent referral for further assessment of the larynx and hypopharynx will be required.
- Globus pharyngeus is common and the 'lump' often disappears during eating.
- Chronic dysphagia caused by neuromuscular disorders may result in aspiration and necessitate a feeding gastrostomy.

Consider referring

- Any patient with true dysphagia requires urgent referral.
- Any patient who has had foreign body sensation lasting for more than 4 weeks (particularly if associated with hoarseness, unilateral otalgia or a neck mass) for which no acute local cause can be found warrants urgent referral.
- Acute dysphagia where the history suggests an ingested foreign body.
- Dysphagia caused by neuromuscular disorders when further investigation or specialist management is needed.
- Patients noted on barium swallow to have a pharyngeal pouch which is producing significant symptoms.

Hoarseness

Most patients presenting with this common symptom will have self-limiting acute laryngitis secondary to an upper respiratory viral infection or recent voice abuse. Hoarseness only becomes of concern when it is not due to such a recognisable cause or when it is prolonged.

Assessment and diagnosis

Is the hoarseness persistent or intermittent? If there is an underlying structural problem (e.g. inflammation, polyp, neoplasia or cord palsy) then the symptom is usually persistent (Table 4.2). In the larger functional group of problems there is no structural pathology and the symptom is often intermittent.

Is the voice gruff or weak? Intrinsic lesions on the vocal cords tend to produce a gruff quality to the voice, whereas a weak voice and a weak-sounding cough (especially in a smoker) suggests a vocal cord palsy.

133

Table 4.2 Classification of organic causes of dysphonia

Inflammatory
- Acute laryngitis (infective)
- Chronic laryngitis

Neoplastic
- Carcinoma of the larynx
- Juvenile laryngeal papillomata

Neurological
- Myasthenia gravis
- Vocal cord paralysis
- Spasmodic dysphonia

Systemic
- Hypothyroidism
- Rheumatoid arthritis

Is there associated dysphagia, stridor or unilateral otalgia? The presence of any of these symptoms would suggest malignant disease of the larynx, hypopharynx or oesophagus.

Is there a history of previous thyroid or cardiothoracic surgery? Such a history might suggest surgical trauma to the vagus nerve (or recurrent laryngeal nerve).

Is the patient myxoedematous? In rare cases hypothyroidism may present with hoarseness.

Is there a history of smoking or voice abuse? These are the commonest factors predisposing to chronic laryngitis.

Is there evidence of disease of the thyroid or lungs? Examination of the thyroid gland and chest (including a chest X-ray if appropriate) is required to exclude a carcinoma at either site, which could result in vocal cord paralysis.

Examinations in the ENT department
Patients with persistent hoarseness lasting for longer than 4 weeks require an examination of the vocal cords to exclude a neoplastic cause. This usually requires referral.

Indirect laryngoscopy: i.e. examination of the larynx with a mirror. This is occasionally difficult (or impossible) because of an active gag reflex.

Fibreoptic laryngoscopy can be performed under local anaesthesia, and is useful if it has proved impossible to examine the larynx with a mirror. It involves passing a 3.5 mm diameter endoscope to the back of the nose and oropharynx in order to visualize the larynx.

Direct laryngoscopy is performed under general anaesthesia, sometimes using microscopic magnification (microlaryngoscopy). As well as allowing visualization of the cords, it also allows biopsy and microsurgical procedures. However, unlike indirect and fibreoptic laryngoscopy, it does not allow assessment of the larynx during phonation, and so it is not a good way of assessing cord movement.

Chronic laryngitis

This is the commonest cause of hoarseness, and the main predisposing factors are smoking and voice abuse. The changes seen in the larynx vary considerably:

- the larynx may appear oedematous or beefy red in colour
- there may be localized vocal cord oedema or vocal cord polyps (Figure 4.12) and these may account for persistent symptoms after the underlying cause has been treated
- singers' nodules (in children they are known as screamers' nodules) may develop bilaterally on the anterior vocal cords and are related to voice trauma (Figure 4.13).

Therapy is aimed at removing or treating the cause, and speech therapy is likely to be helpful. Laryngeal microsurgery may have a part to play in a small number of patients, especially if they have associated vocal cord polyps or nodules.

Neoplasia

Benign neoplasia: juvenile laryngeal papillomatosis is caused by the human papilloma virus. In children it initially presents with

135

hoarseness but may eventually cause stridor and airways obstruction. Single papillomata may occur in adults.

Malignant neoplasia: squamous cell carcinoma of the larynx (Figure 4.14) is the commonest form of head and neck cancer. It arises almost invariably in smokers and although formerly much more common in men, the sex incidence is changing as more women smoke. Direct laryngoscopy is required to obtain a histological diagnosis.

Treatment in a large number of cases will be with primary radiotherapy. Surgery in the form of a laryngectomy is in the majority of cases reserved for patients in whom radiotherapy has failed.

Vocal cord paralysis

This can be caused by any lesion along the course of the vagus nerve from its origin in the posterior fossa through the neck and chest (on the left side) to the larynx. The common causes of a vocal cord palsy include:

■ neoplasm (carcinoma of the bronchus, oesophagus or thyroid, skull base tumours)

■ iatrogenic causes (surgical trauma in thyroid and cardiothoracic surgery)

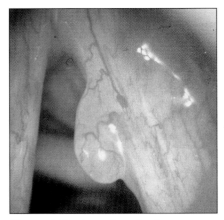
Figure 4.12 *A vocal cord polyp.*

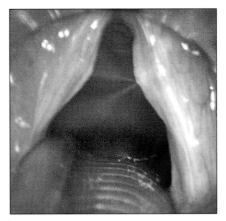
Figure 4.13 *Vocal cord nodules.*

- idiopathic causes (many patients fall into this group after investigations identify no underlying pathology to account for the palsy).

If a cause for the palsy is identified this is managed appropriately. If no cause is identified, in the majority of patients the hoarseness will resolve over 6–12 months, either because of recovery of the palsy or due to compensatory movement of the other cord.

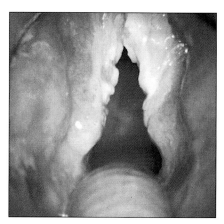

Figure 4.14 *Carcinoma of the vocal cord.*

If no recovery is seen over a 6-month period, surgery can be undertaken to improve the strength and quality of the voice. This can be achieved endoscopically using a Teflon injection to displace the paralysed cord towards the midline (i.e. to move it closer to the mobile opposite cord) or as an open operation (thyroplasty, which can be performed under local anaesthetic).

Key points

- If there is a structural cause for hoarseness the symptom is usually persistent.
- If there is a functional cause for hoarseness the symptom is often intermittent.
- Vocal cord palsy tends to produce a weak voice rather than a gruff one.
- Myxoedema may present with hoarseness.
- Any patient with persistent hoarseness (greater than 4 weeks) will require an examination of the vocal cords to exclude a neoplastic cause and this will usually require referral.

- Diagnosis rests primarily on the clinical examination (either indirect or fibreoptic laryngoscopy).
- Malignant laryngeal tumours are usually managed by radiotherapy, with surgery used for radiotherapy failures.

Consider referring

- Any adult with hoarseness lasting for longer than 4 weeks should be referred for an examination of the larynx.
- Any patient with hoarseness who has associated dysphagia (or foreign body sensation in the throat), stridor or unilateral otalgia where the ear appears normal on examination.
- Any patient with hoarseness and a history of previous thyroid or cardiothoracic surgery.

Stridor

Stridor is noisy breathing resulting from upper airway obstruction. A narrowing at the level of the larynx or trachea causes inspiratory stridor, in contrast to bronchial narrowing which causes an expiratory wheeze.

Adults rarely present with stridor (Table 4.3). It is more common in children because their airways are of relatively small diameter, and their laryngeal cartilages may be soft and collapsible.

Laryngotracheobronchitis (croup)

The vast majority of children presenting with stridor will have laryngotracheobronchitis (croup). The child will often have a preceding history of an upper respiratory tract infection and will develop a 'barking' cough. The physiological changes that occur in the upper airway during sleep mean that any stridor is most likely to

Table 4.3 Age-specific causes of stridor

Neonates	Children	Adults
■ Congenital tumours or cysts	■ Laryngotracheo-bronchitis (croup)	■ Laryngeal cancer
■ Webs	■ Epiglottitis/supraglottitis	■ Laryngeal trauma
■ Laryngomalacia	■ Acute laryngitis	■ Acute laryngitis
■ Subglottic stenosis	■ Foreign body	■ Epiglottitis/supraglottitis
	■ Retropharyngeal abscess	
	■ Respiratory papillomata	

occur when the child is asleep, and any daytime stridor may therefore be an indication for hospital admission.

Treatment: croup is caused by viral infection and so antibiotics are not indicated, particularly as the fear of Haemophilus-related epiglottitis has diminished as a result of the routine immunization of children against *Haemophilus influenzae* B infections.

The mainstay of the treatment of the stridor caused by croup is initially steam inhalation (the parent being instructed to sit the child in the kitchen and to fill the room with steam) over 10–20 minutes. If this fails to settle the stridor then an inhaled steroid (Pulmicort via nebulizer and mask) is required.

Most children will improve with such treatment and will not require hospital referral. In the majority of children with croup the stridor tends to be troublesome for 1–2 nights only. If the stridor is severe and fails to settle with standard treatment, then urgent hospital admission for nursing with humidification and oxygen is necessary.

Acute epiglottitis

This is a potentially life-threatening condition which can come on over a few hours and is caused by infection with *Haemophilus influenzae* B. (Thankfully with routine Hib immunization of children the incidence of this condition in the UK is decreasing.) The child is clearly very unwell with fever, severe respiratory distress and severe stridor. The child tends to sit up rather than lie down, and may drool saliva.

The child's throat should not be examined as this could potentially precipitate upper airway obstruction.

Steam inhalations and nebulized steroids will not help. Urgent hospital admission is indicated for treatment with parenteral antibiotics and, in some cases, endotracheal intubation.

Laryngomalacia

This condition is characterized by a 'floppy larynx'. The cartilaginous framework of the larynx can collapse with the negative pressure of inspiration, producing stridor, especially during exertion or on crying. The stridor is often positional, being worse when lying on the back and better when lying on the front (when the tongue falls forward taking the epiglottis with it and improving the airway). As the vocal cords are normal, the cry is normal.

In the majority of children laryngomalacia is self-limiting, resolving by the age of 3–4 years. As the stridor is intermittent referral need not be on an urgent basis.

Congenital abnormalities

Congential abnormalities causing stridor in children include subglottic haemangioma, webs and subglottic stenosis.

Laryngeal web between the anterior vocal cords is one of the commonest congenital abnormalities and can cause recurrent stridor, particularly when the child has upper respiratory infections. As the child and the larynx grow bigger, so the web is stretched, and usually disappears by the age of 4–5 years.

Subglottic stenosis may be congenital, or may be acquired in cases of trauma or prolonged endotracheal intubation (particularly likely in premature babies).

Foreign bodies

The child will be well one minute and stridulous the next. Often — but not always — this occurs while the child is eating. If the child is small enough, he or she may be held upside down by the feet and given a slap on the back. In older children the Heimlich manoeuvre should be used. If neither are successful then the foreign body may need to be removed endoscopically.

Laryngeal papillomata

These are akin to warts in the larynx. They initially lead to a change in cry/voice but eventually may produce stridor. Treatment involves endoscopic surgical removal using a laser.

Stridor in adults

Causes of stridor in adults include epiglottitis, laryngeal cancer and laryngeal trauma.

Epiglottitis or supraglottitis is occasionally seen in adults, and pain is a more prominent symptom than stridor. Parenteral antibiotics are usually indicated.

Laryngeal trauma: injuries to the larynx are usually produced when the laryngeal framework is crushed against the cervical vertebrae in road traffic accidents or as the result of a kick or blow. Haematoma and swelling occur as a result of tears in the laryngeal mucosa and cause stridor.

Management in the ENT department

All patients presenting with persisting or recurrent stridor (other than croup) will need referral so that the larynx can be visualized.

If the stridor is both persistent and severe then at the least the patient requires observation in hospital.

When severe stridor is present there is a possibility of complete upper respiratory obstruction. Any one of the following procedures may be required, depending on where the emergency occurs and the experience of the doctor concerned.

Laryngotomy involves placing a wide bore needle or knife through the cricothyroid membrane (between the cricoid and thyroid cartilages) and keeping the hole open. This is probably the most appropriate treatment for emergencies outside a hospital setting.

Endotracheal intubation is usually the most appropriate treatment within a hospital. However, it may be difficult or impossible in laryngeal trauma, or when a large laryngeal/pharyngeal tumour is the cause of the upper airway obstruction. If a foreign body is the cause of the problem, it may be seen and removed at the time of passing the tube.

Tracheostomy is performed if it proves impossible to intubate the patient.

If none of these procedures is immediately required, the patient will be monitored closely in hospital as the clinical condition can rapidly deteriorate.

Key points

■ Stridor can be life-threatening and management often takes precedence over diagnosis.
■ Children are particularly at risk because of the relatively small size of their airways.
■ Acute epiglottitis in children can be life-threatening — the presence of drooling in an extremely sick child suggests epiglottitis rather than croup.

- Stridor in adults rarely progresses as rapidly as in children.
- Suspect an inhaled foreign body in a previously well child who develops abrupt wheezing or stridor.

Consider referring

- Any child with persistent stridor needs urgent referral.
- Any adult with persisting stridor needs a formal ENT assessment, even if it is not required as a matter of urgency.

Neck lumps

Family practitioners may discover neck lumps when examining patients, or may be asked for advice by patients who themselves have found single or multiple neck lumps. The following normal structures in the neck are often discovered by patients, causing them alarm and precipitating consultation with their doctors:

- prominent carotid bifurcation
- submandibular glands
- hyoid bone
- jugulodigastric lymph node in anterior triangle
- transverse process of axis (between mastoid process and angle of mandible).

History
How quickly did the swelling appear, and does it hurt? It is important to establish the speed of onset and presence or absence of pain. A sudden painful swelling strongly suggests an inflammatory condition, whereas a slowly-progressive, non-painful swelling is more suggestive of a neoplastic pathology.

Did the appearance of the neck lump coincide with associated symptoms of an upper respiratory tract infection? Acute inflammatory lymph node swelling associated with infection of the nose, throat, mouth or ear is the commonest cause of neck lumps in both children and adults.

Is there more than one lump? Multiple lumps are probably lymph nodes.

Is the swelling in the midline? The commonest midline swellings include:

■ thyroid lumps, which move vertically on swallowing
■ thyroglossal cyst, usually at about the level of the thyroid or hyoid cartilage, which moves on swallowing and on protruding the tongue
■ dermoid cyst, which usually arises above the hyoid bone — there is often a swelling in the floor of the mouth pushing the tongue upwards as well as an external swelling.

Are there any associated symptoms suggesting a primary head and neck site of malignancy? For example:

■ dysphagia (pharynx/oesophagus)
■ dysphonia (larynx/hypopharynx)
■ nasal symptoms (nasopharynx).

Examination and investigations

It is important to perform a thorough examination of the head and neck. The scalp should be examined to exclude an inflammatory condition or a primary skin cancer in this area. The ears, nose, mouth and throat must be thoroughly examined to exclude inflammatory or malignant conditions. The neck is best examined while standing behind the patient.

Multiple lumps are most likely to be lymph nodes. In this case evidence of lymphadenopathy at other sites should be sought, and the liver and spleen assessed.

A full blood count, monospot blood test or chest X-ray may be appropriate.

Assessment in the ENT department

Patients will be given a full ENT examination including endoscopic examination of the nose, postnasal space, hypopharynx and larynx. Fine-needle aspiration cytology may also be performed, and a CT or MRI scan carried out.

If no diagnosis can be made from these investigations, the patient will be admitted for an endoscopic examination of the upper aerodigestive tract under general anaesthesia (panendoscopy).

The lump will be excised for histological diagnosis only if the investigations revealed no underlying primary carcinoma.

Paediatric neck lumps

It is normal for children to have easily palpable neck lymph nodes.

Midline lumps: the commonest midline mass in children is a thyroglossal cyst (Figure 4.15) located below the hyoid bone. More rarely a dermoid cyst may present as a submental swelling located above the hyoid.

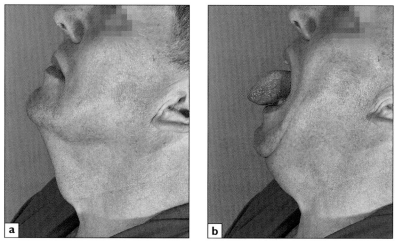

Figure 4.15 *A thyroglossal cyst (a): it moves when the patient protrudes the tongue (b).*

Lateral lumps may be inflammatory, congenital or neoplastic.

■ Inflammatory lumps: the vast majority of pathological neck lumps seen in children presenting in family practice are associated with infection in the head and neck. The lumps are multiple, bilateral and tender. They are self-limiting and usually settle in 4–6 weeks.

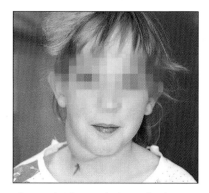

Figure 4.16 *A right branchial cyst.*

■ Congenital lumps: most solitary lateral neck masses in children are congenital in origin. They include cystic hygromas and — more commonly — branchial cysts (Figure 4.16), which present as a tense, fluctuant swelling postero-inferior to the angle of the mandible that does not move on swallowing.

■ Neoplastic lumps: neoplasia in children is usually due to primary cancer in the neck (e.g. lymphoma, neuroblastoma, rhabdomyosarcoma).

Adult neck lumps

Midline lumps: the commonest midline neck lump in adults is of thyroid origin.

Lateral lumps: as in children, lateral lumps in adults may be inflammatory, neoplastic or congenital.

■ Inflammatory lumps: the vast majority of neck lumps seen in adults presenting in family practice are associated with acute head and neck infection/inflammation. As in children, the lumps are bilateral and tender, and are associated with clear evidence of the primary infection. Almost all such cases will resolve in 4–6 weeks. If they fail to do so, referral for assessment is advisable, although even then most will only show reactive lymph node changes.

■ Neoplastic lumps: any firm, painless, lateral neck lump appearing in an adult (especially if over 40 years of age) that is not associated with an acute infection should be treated as metastatic cancer (Figure 4.17) until proven otherwise. It may be the first sign of malignant disease and the primary is usually above the clavicles. Clearly such cases should be referred for ENT assessment to exclude squamous cell carcinoma. If the lump is below the ear lobule, and behind the ramus and angle of the mandible, it may be arising within the parotid gland (Figure 4.18). If this is the case, it is again more likely to be neoplastic, although the most common neoplasm in the parotid is the benign pleomorphic adenoma. Malignant parotid tumours may be associated with pain and facial weakness.

■ Congenital lumps: although branchial cysts are congenital in origin, they sometimes do not present until adult life.

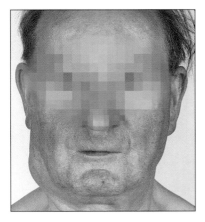

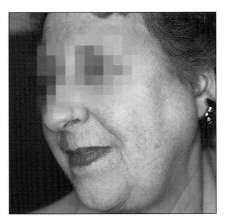

Figure 4.17 *A large cervical lymph node in a patient with carcinoma of the hypopharynx.*

Figure 4.18 *Characteristic site of parotid mass.*

Key points

- Patients are often alarmed when they palpate normal structures in the neck.
- It is normal for children to have easily palpable lymph nodes.
- Multiple, tender neck lumps of sudden onset are probably cervical lymphadenopathy associated with head and neck infection.
- Slowly-progressive, firm, painless lateral neck swelling may be the first sign of malignant disease.
- The commonest midline neck lump in children is a thyroglossal cyst.
- The commonest isolated lateral neck lump in children is a branchial cyst.
- In adults endoscopy of the upper aerodigestive tract is mandatory to exclude a primary squamous cell carcinoma in the area before considering an excision biopsy.

Consider referring

- Any patient with a persisting neck mass where there is no history to suggest an inflammatory cause.
- Any patient with a neck mass and persisting dysphagia, dysphonia or nasal symptoms.
- Any patient with a neck lump which persists for more than 6 weeks (even if it is initially associated with an inflammatory cause).

Chapter 5

Injuries, emergencies and mandatory referrals

Trauma to the ear

Injuries to the pinna

Auricular haematoma (Figure 5.1): blunt trauma may produce bleeding deep to the perichondrium, which is stripped from the underlying cartilage so that the ear becomes swollen and the normal folds of the pinna are lost. As the cartilage depends on the perichondrium for its blood supply, the haematoma will lead to necrosis of the cartilage and result in a cauliflower ear unless it is drained adequately.

The haematoma should be aspirated, a pressure bandage applied, and the patient reviewed in 2 days. Referral for incision and drainage is required

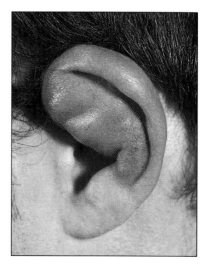

Figure 5.1 *Auricular haematoma.*

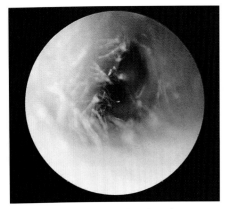

Figure 5.2 *A metallic bead in the ear canal.*

if aspiration is unsuccessful or if the haematoma recurs.

The external ear canal

Foreign bodies often find their way into the ear canal (Figure 5.2) and can be difficult to remove.

Syringing should only be attempted if the tympanic membrane is intact, and this should be carefully checked. Syringing is sometimes successful for non-vegetable foreign bodies (vegetable materials tend to swell when wet); insects may be drowned with olive oil and then removed by syringing.

If the foreign body is not readily removable then referral (nearly always non-urgent) is advisable as there is a danger of pushing the object further into the ear canal. It is also wise to refer cases where associated trauma to the tympanic membrane is suspected, or if there is risk of damage to the tympanic membrane when removing the foreign body.

In the ENT department, foreign body removal is facilitated by the use of an operating microscope or headlight. If the object is soft, crocodile or Tilley's forceps will be used; a hook or Jobson Horne probe will be used if the object is solid. Despite these aids, children may still require general anaesthesia to allow foreign bodies to be removed.

Injuries to the external meatus are almost exclusively related to insertion of cotton buds, hairgrips, pencils, etc. The result is a laceration of the canal wall with resulting bleeding, usually requiring no active treatment. The external auditory canal is often full of dry blood and no attempt should be made to remove this. The results of Rinne and Weber tuning fork tests should be recorded (normal tests suggest that the ossicular chain is intact) and the patient reviewed one week later.

Referral for further evaluation (usually on a non-urgent basis) may be necessary if there is any possibility that either the tympanic membrane or ossicular chain is injured. If the patient has a perforation of the eardrum and normal tuning fork tests, it is entirely reasonable to wait for 2–4 weeks for the perforation to heal: if the hearing is then normal, no referral is necessary.

Injuries to the middle and inner ear

Blast injuries: the most common blast-type injury seen in family practice is caused by a simple slap across the face. The typical injury produced is a tear in the tympanic membrane, but it may be difficult to view the eardrum because of blood in the canal. The Rinne test may be negative and the Weber may lateralise to the affected side. The patient should be advised to keep the ear dry and to report any discharge. There is no indication for the routine use of antibiotics in the absence of evidence of infection. The vast majority of these injuries will heal spontaneously over 2–4 weeks, and referral is not necessary.

In more severe blast injuries (e.g. those caused by explosions), rupture of the tympanic membrane may be accompanied by damage to the cochlea, resulting in sensorineural hearing loss and tinnitus. Imbalance may occur if the vestibular function of the inner ear is affected. In such cases it is important to check for the following:

- nystagmus
- cerebrospinal fluid (CSF) otorrhoea (dipstick positive for glucose)
- facial nerve palsy
- Weber lateralising to the opposite ear (indicating sensorineural hearing loss).

Referral of these more severe injuries is clearly appropriate.

Otitic barotrauma: this condition is seen when the ambient pressure is rising, e.g. when scuba diving or descending in an aircraft. It can produce otalgia with some extravasation of blood into the layers of the eardrum or middle ear (haemotympanum). In severe cases the eardrum may rupture. The vast majority of cases resolve spontaneously, although this may take some weeks.

Occasionally the barotrauma is great enough to cause rupture of the inner ear membranes (perilymph fistula) resulting in:

- sensorineural hearing loss
- vertigo with nystagmus
- tinnitus.

In these circumstances urgent referral is clearly indicated.

Head injuries: severe head injuries may be associated with temporal bone fractures, which in turn may be associated with:

- blood in the external canal
- CSF otorrhoea
- haemotympanum
- hearing loss (sensorineural through damage to the cochlea, conductive through disruption of the middle ear/ossicular chain)
- facial paralysis.

Total facial paralysis immediately following injury suggests major injury to the nerve (which may warrant surgical exploration), whereas delayed paralysis usually recovers spontaneously.

Any patient with any of the above symptoms and a history of head injury warrants urgent referral for further assessment.

Key points

- An auricular haematoma requires aspiration, or incision and drainage.
- For non-vegetable foreign bodies in the ear canal syringing is sometimes successful, providing that the tympanic membrane

is definitely intact.

- A traumatic perforation of the eardrum following a slap on the ear is likely to heal spontaneously without the need for prophylactic antibiotics.
- Otitic barotrauma is likely to settle spontaneously.
- Any patient with bleeding from the ear, CSF otorrhoea, hearing loss or facial weakness following a head injury should be suspected of having a temporal bone fracture.

Consider referring

- Any patient with an auricular haematoma in whom either aspiration is unsuccessful or the haematoma recurs after aspiration.
- Any patient (especially a child) with a foreign body in the ear canal that is not readily removable.
- Any patient with sensorineural hearing loss, tinnitus or vertigo (i.e. evidence of cochlear damage) following a blast injury.
- Any patient with a history of barotrauma leading to sudden hearing loss, tinnitus and vertigo.
- Any patient with bleeding from the ear, CSF otorrhoea, hearing loss or facial weakness following a head injury.

Trauma to the nose

Nasal fractures

Trauma to the nose occurs for many reasons — the nasal bones are the most commonly fractured bones in the human body — and mainly affects young males. If the blow comes from the side, the nasal bones are deviated (Figure 5.3); if the blow comes from the front, the nasal bones are often depressed.

The patient presents with:
- soft tissue swelling over the nose and maxilla
- nasal obstruction and bleeding
- nasal deformity.

The following should also be considered:
- septal haematoma
- CSF leak
- other associated facial fractures.

Nasal deformity: initially the deformity may not be obvious because of associated soft tissue swelling, in which case the patient should be reviewed 5–7 days after the injury. If referral is necessary (i.e. if residual deformity is suspected) then the patient should be sent to the ENT department approximately one week after the injury occurred.

Septal haematoma: the nasal septum is grossly widened and feels 'boggy' if touched with a probe (unlike a deviated septum which is hard). The haematoma often blocks both sides of the nose completely. The blood strips the muco-perichondrium from the septal cartilage, from which it receives its blood supply. If this is uncorrected, devitalization and necrosis of the underlying cartilage occurs, and the nose subsequently collapses. If the haematoma becomes infected then septal collapse is also highly likely. Treatment is by surgical drainage and appropriate antibiotic therapy: referral is mandatory.

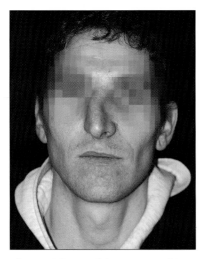

Figure 5.3 *Nasal fracture resulting in external deformity.*

Treatment in the ENT department: radiography is not

essential for an isolated nasal fracture in terms of clinical management (any deformity is assessed clinically).

The decision to reduce the fracture is made on the appearance of the nose once the soft tissue swelling settles, and the fracture can be reduced about 10 days after the injury (i.e. after the swelling has settled and before the fracture becomes too fixed by healing).

Simple fractures may be reduced under local or general anaesthetic. More complex fractures occasionally require more active surgical treatment, including wiring to maintain an unstable fracture.

Foreign bodies

Small children (and occasionally psychologically-disturbed adults) insert objects into their noses. Many children are seen in family practice before they develop symptoms — the parents may have seen the child inserting the foreign body or may have noticed the object if it is visible in the nostril. A long-standing foreign body presents with a unilateral mucopurulent discharge from the child's nose (Figure 5.4).

If confident of being able to remove the foreign body, the family practitioner may attempt this using a blunt hook. However, the child will usually only tolerate one such attempt without a general anaesthetic. Urgent referral is therefore advisable if there is any doubt about removing the object on the first try, as there is a risk of the child inhaling it into the lower airway.

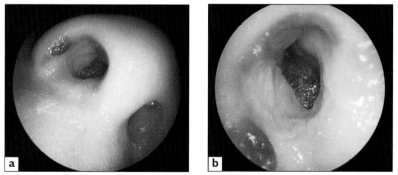

Figure 5.4 *(a) View of foreign body in right nasal cavity. Note excoriation of nasal vestibule. (b) Endoscopic view of foreign body (piece of sponge) in right nasal cavity.*

155

Treatment in the ENT department: if initial attempts at extracting the foreign body are unsuccessful it will be removed under a general anaesthetic.

Key points

- Patients with nasal fractures with obvious deformity should be sent to the ENT department for assessment approximately one week after the injury occurred.
- A patient with a nasal fracture with an associated septal haematoma requires urgent referral.
- Collapse of the nose (saddle deformity) can follow an untreated nasal septal haematoma.
- Nasal fractures are reduced about 10 days after the injury.
- A long-standing foreign body is the most frequent cause of a unilateral mucopurulent discharge from a child's nose.

Consider referring

- Any patient with a nasal fracture and associated nasal deformity.
- Any patient with a nasal fracture and associated complications (e.g. septal haematoma).
- Any patient suspected of having a septal haematoma requires urgent referral.
- Any child with a unilateral nasal discharge.

Trauma to the throat

Trauma in this area may be external (a sharp or a blunt injury), or it may involve inhaled or swallowed foreign bodies.

External trauma

In a sharp injury (e.g. after a knifing) the edges of the lacerations are clean-cut and bony damage is unusual. In a blunt injury lacerations tend to be ragged and fractures of the cartilages of the larynx and trachea may occur.

The two significant areas of injury are the carotid sheath (where injury kills by blood loss) and the larynx/trachea (where injury kills by airway obstruction).

Initial assessment: assessment of any patient who has suffered trauma to the throat initially involves ensuring that there is no respiratory difficulty, and treating any bleeding and airway obstruction. The following points should then be considered.

- What is the voice like? A fractured or injured larynx will cause hoarseness. Flattening of the larynx (loss of the Adam's apple prominence) could indicate a fracture, as could the presence of surgical emphysema within the neck.

- Is breathing difficult? This could be the direct effect of injury to the upper airway or could be related to a pressure effect on the airway by bleeding within the neck.

- Is it sore or difficult to swallow? Pain on swallowing suggests significant laryngeal trauma, e.g. fracture of laryngeal cartilages.

Assessment and management in the ENT department: plain radiographs may be helpful in confirming the presence of air in the soft tissues. Indirect laryngoscopy or flexible nasolaryngoscopy will be performed in all patients, to assess the damage to the larynx and the safety of the airway. If a laryngeal fracture is suspected, the neck will probably need to be explored.

Management is directed to ensuring that the patient is not in respiratory difficulty and that any severe bleeding has stopped. If the airway needs to be protected then intubation is preferred to tracheostomy.

Inhaled foreign bodies

These are most frequently seen in children. As impaction in the larynx may be rapidly fatal, the Heimlich manoeuvre should be attempted. It is, however, more common for the foreign body to lodge beyond the larynx where it may produce little in the way of symptoms in the short term.

Assessment: there is usually an initial episode of choking and coughing, but thereafter the patient may have little in the way of symptoms. The diagnosis of an inhaled foreign body should always be considered in a child with a history of choking/coughing who then develops unilateral chest signs. A chest X-ray may show signs of hyperinflation or collapse, but foreign bodies are often not radio-opaque.

Management in the ENT department: all foreign bodies, once detected, should be removed immediately endoscopically under general anaesthesia.

Swallowed foreign bodies

Children will swallow anything (Figure 5.5), but in adults the problem is usually caused by food impaction, e.g. bones or badly chewed meat (food bolus obstruction).

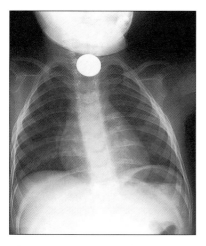

Figure 5.5 *Ingested radio-opaque foreign body on a plain radiograph.*

Assessment and localization: most patients give a reliable history of foreign body ingestion. Unfortunately, it is often difficult for the patient to differentiate between an object that remains lodged and one that has passed on. In the latter case symptoms persist (possibly because of mucosal trauma of some kind) but improve over the course of a few days. If the foreign body is still lodged, symptoms will become worse over this period.

If the foreign body is lodged in the mouth or oropharynx (as is often the case with a fish bone), localization is possible, with the patient able to point to the side affected. An impacted foreign body in the pharyngo-oesophagus will pro-duce less accurate localization but more often acute dysphagia with difficulty in swallowing even saliva.

Assessment and management in the ENT department: most foreign bodies in the mouth and oropharynx can be seen with a light source and tongue depressor.

If the object is lodged in the pharyngo-oesophagus, then a mirror and headlight will be required to perform indirect laryngoscopy, or a flexible nasolaryngoscope can be used. With these techniques, either the foreign body itself will be seen, or a build-up of saliva (pooling of saliva) secondary to the distal obstruction observed.

Soft tissue neck X-rays together with a chest X-ray may help localize a foreign body, especially if it is radio-opaque. Occasionally screening with a contrast medium (barium swallow) may be justified, particularly if an oesophageal perforation is suspected in association with the foreign body.

If there is no definite history of bone ingestion (and hence less likelihood of perforation), it may be reasonable to wait for 24 hours in the hope that the foreign body (e.g. food bolus obstruction) will pass spontaneously. Muscle relaxants may be given in the hope of increasing this possibility.

Removal of fish bones lodged in the tongue base/tonsil can often be achieved in a co-operative patient without resorting to general anaesthesia. Bones lodged in the pharyngo-oesophagus will require endoscopic removal under general anaesthesia.

Key points

- Assessment of any patient who has suffered trauma to the throat initially involves treatment of any bleeding and airway obstruction. If the airway needs to be protected intubation is preferred to tracheostomy.
- The diagnosis of an inhaled foreign body should always be considered in a child with a history of choking/coughing who develops unilateral chest signs.
- When a foreign body has been swallowed it is often difficult for the patient to differentiate between an object that remains lodged and one that has passed on.
- If a swallowed foreign body is lodged in the mouth or oropharynx (often the case with fish bones), localization is possible with the patient able to point to the side affected.
- An impacted foreign body in the pharyngo-oesophagus will produce less accurate localization but more often acute dysphagia.

Consider referring

- Any patient who has suffered a penetrating neck injury.
- Any patient who has suffered a blunt neck injury who has any symptoms that suggest laryngeal injury/fracture.
- Any child with a history of choking/coughing who was thought to have something in the mouth at the time the symptoms began.
- Any patient with a history of foreign body ingestion who has associated dysphagia which is not improving.
- Any patient with a history of foreign body ingestion and symptoms suggestive of perforation (chest pain, dyspnoea).

Danger signs and symptoms in ENT

It is impossible to provide a list of signs and symptoms which in isolation warrant mandatory referral. As in every aspect of clinical life in family practice, there has to be a large element of common sense. This section aims to give some help to the practitioner who has to try to assess whether symptoms or signs may signify some serious underlying pathology in the ear (Table 5.1), nose (Table 5.2) and throat (Table 5.3).

As a general principle, if symptoms are unilateral they should be taken more seriously.

Table 5.1 Danger signs and symptoms in the ear

Sign/symptom	Comments	Possible diagnosis
Unilateral deafness/asymmetric deafness	If sensorineural in nature needs further investigation	Acoustic neuroma
Unilateral deafness	If conductive hearing loss secondary to middle ear effusion in an adult (not following URTI)	Carcinoma of postnasal space
Unilateral tinnitus	If no identifiable outer/middle ear pathology, then requires investigation	Acoustic neuroma
Unilateral otalgia	If ear looks normal, assume referred pain	Malignant disease of the oral cavity, oropharynx, hypopharynx, larynx
Smelly otorrhoea	Perforation in the attic/posterosuperior part of eardrum	Cholesteatoma until proved otherwise

Table 5.2 Danger signs and symptoms in the nose

Sign/symptom	Comments	Possible diagnosis
Unilateral nasal discharge in a child	Unilateral rhinorrhoea is unusual	Foreign body until proved otherwise
Unilateral, blood-stained discharge in an adolescent	Angiofibroma is rare but any history of epistaxis/nasal obstruction in this age group should be taken seriously	Angiofibroma (benign locally aggressive tumour) until proved otherwise
Unilateral blood-stained discharge in an adult	Especially if associated with facial swelling/epiphora	Malignant tumour of the nose/paranasal sinuses
Proptosis	Always requires investigation	Local causes include sino-nasal neoplasm
Unilateral polyp	Simple inflammatory polyps are usually bilateral	Neoplastic nasal polyp until proved otherwise

Table 5.3 Danger signs and symptoms in the throat

Sign/symptom	Comments	Possible diagnosis
Hoarseness	Any adult with hoarseness for more than 4 weeks requires referral	Carcinoma of larynx
Dysphagia	Any patient with true dysphagia (as opposed to a foreign body sensation) warrants urgent referral	Carcinoma of pharyngo-oesophagus
Haemoptysis	Usually associated with bronchogenic carcinoma, but may be seen in carcinoma of upper aero-digestive tract	Carcinoma of upper aero-digestive tract
Lump in neck	Any lateral neck lump in an adult is metastatic carcinoma until proved otherwise	Secondary lymph node involvement from carcinoma of upper aero-digestive tract
Unilateral tonsillar enlargement	There is often some asymmetry of the tonsils, but if marked it often warrants referral	Tonsillar lymphoma
Stridor	Any patient with persistent stridor requires urgent referral	Many possible diagnoses – all may precipitate life-threatening upper airway obstruction

Head and neck cancer

Head and neck cancer is one of the more uncommon cancers, accounting for some 4% of new cases. In the UK the incidence is approximately 12 per 100,000, and it is the eighth most common cancer in men and the sixteenth most common in women. The term encompasses a wide range of malignant tumours, but the majority are squamous carcinomas that arise from the mucosa of the upper aero-digestive tract.

The most influential aetiological factor in cancer of the head and neck is smoking tobacco: up to 90% of patients with cancer of the oral cavity, oropharynx, hypopharynx or larynx have a history of smoking.

The functional and psychological effects of head and neck cancer are greater than those found in many other forms of malignancy, and may involve changes in swallowing, speech, respiration, hearing and sight, as well as obvious changes in appearance.

The 5-year mortality rates from head and neck cancer remain one of the highest for any cancer, in spite of advances in radiotherapy and surgery that have certainly helped to achieve better local control of the disease and improved quality of life for the patients. Despite this depressing picture, there is a wide variation in prognosis with early cancers of the larynx having a cure rate of 90–95% with radical radiotherapy. The poor prognosis for many of these tumours is related to the late onset of symptoms and — in some cases — patient delay in presentation.

The summary of the presenting features of individual head and neck cancers given here (Table 5.4) is intended to help to lead to the earlier diagnosis of these tumours. They are listed in order of decreasing incidence, beginning with laryngeal cancer, which is the most common.

Table 5.4 Head and neck cancers

Cancer site	Symptoms of primary	Symptoms of spread beyond primary site
Larynx	■ Hoarseness ■ Dysphagia ■ Stridor	■ Neck lump ■ Otalgia
Oral cavity	■ Ulcer ■ Difficulty with chewing, swallowing and speech	■ Neck lump ■ Otalgia

Pharynx
■ Nasopharynx
	■ Nasal obstruction
	■ Epistaxis
	■ Unilateral glue ear (common in Chinese)
		■ Neck lump
		■ Cranial neuropathy
		  −V: pain/paraesthesia
		  − III, IV, VI: diplopia
		  − X, XII: dysphagia

■ Oropharynx	■ Ulcer ■ Sore throat ■ Dysphagia ■ Foreign body sensation	■ Neck lump ■ Otalgia ■ Trismus
■ Hypopharynx	■ Sore throat ■ Dysphagia ■ Foreign body sensation ■ Hoarseness	■ Neck lump ■ Otalgia

Table 5.4 Continued

Sino-nasal

- Nose
  - Obstruction
  - Discharge

  - Neck lump
  - Trismus
  - Facial swelling
- Eye
  - Proptosis
  - Epiphora
  - Diplopia

  - Paraesthesia

- Mouth
  - Loose teeth
  - Palatal ulcer/swelling

Parotid
- Lump
- VII weakness
- Pain

  - Associated lymphadenopathy
  - Skin induration
  - Trismus

Ear canal/middle ear
- Bloody otorrhoea
- Pain
- VII weakness
- Hearing loss

  - Neck lumps

Chapter 6

Practical procedures in family practice

Several practical procedures that are useful in the management of simple ENT problems can be performed safely in family practice. Their use can reduce the necessity for referral for specialist management.

The ear

Removing wax

If wax is lying within the superficial part of the ear canal and is of a suitable consistency, then with a good light source and instrumentation (a wax hook is useful) the wax can be removed, taking care not to scratch the sensitive skin.

Hard impacted wax may need to be softened with topical ceruminolytic ear drops (olive oil or sodium bicarbonate) before removal. Failure to remove the wax should not create despondency — even an otolaryngologist will have difficulty with this approach at times, and will resort to the use of the microscope and suction in the outpatient department.

Syringing the ear canal will clear the wax in the majority of cases. The canal is straightened by pulling the pinna posterosuperiorly and the water jet (tap water at body temperature) should be aimed at the roof of the ear canal. The canal and eardrum must be examined afterwards. Waterproof clothing for the patient is essential.

Syringing is contraindicated in:

- only-hearing ear
- history of perforation
- previous ear surgery
- recent trauma.

Dry-mopping the discharging ear

A large part of the management of the discharging ear involves clearing the ear canal of debris. Commercial cotton buds are usually too bulky, and cotton wool wound onto a Jobson Horne probe or orange stick is preferable. This can be used to mop away the excess discharge visible at the lateral end of the ear canal.

Inserting an ear wick

If the ear canal in otitis externa is very narrow or occluded, then topical drops will not penetrate to the canal. In these circumstances the use of an otowick is simple and effective. Before insertion it is firm and narrow, and easy to insert into the canal. When drops are applied it softens and expands, and may be left for several days (the patient should continue to use the drops) until the ear canal oedema has settled and the canal has opened.

Removing a foreign body

Syringing: the majority of foreign bodies (other than vegetable matter which may swell if exposed to water) can be removed by syringing.

Using instruments: appropriate instruments and a good light source are essential. The method of instrumental removal depends on the type of foreign body — a pair of crocodile forceps can grasp cotton wool, paper and pieces of foam. Forceps should not be used to grasp a smooth round object (e.g. a bead) as it is likely to spring out of the jaws and end up even further within the meatus. A blunt hook may be inserted beyond the object (if it is not impacted) and then gently pulled out.

Referral: young children may not lie still for objects to be removed with an instrument, and they may not co-operate with syringing. In such cases (or if appropriate instruments and lighting are not available) referral is wise.

The nose

Removing a foreign body
The child should be asked to blow his or her nose to see if the foreign body will dislodge. If this is unsuccessful and the foreign body is visible, it is likely to be lying on the floor of the nose between the inferior turbinate and septum.
- If the object is *soft*, removal is best achieved with a pair of fine forceps.
- If the object is *hard*, a blunt hook should be passed beyond the object, which is then pulled out.

Nasal cautery
The most convenient way of achieving this is with chemical cautery with silver nitrate sticks. The procedure is only appropriate for an anterior source of bleeding: posterior bleeds are inaccessible as far as cautery is concerned unless a microscope or endoscope is employed. Chemical cautery in the face of brisk active bleeding is unlikely to arrest the bleeding, and there is a risk that the chemical will be washed onto the skin of the nasal vestibule/upper lip by the flow of blood (creating a skin burn which may produce permanent scarring). For the recurrent epistaxes seen in children cautery is usually effective in reducing the frequency of the bleeds.

169

Silver nitrate cautery is therefore most likely to be employed in children with a history of recurrent anterior epistaxes who are not actively bleeding when seen. In this situation anterior rhinoscopy often reveals prominent vessels on the anterior nasal septum. If these are seen then the following procedure should be followed.

- Place cotton wool soaked in 4% lignocaine (adding a small amount of 1:1000 adrenaline produces useful vasoconstriction) in the affected nostril and leave for 5 minutes. Cautery without anaesthesia is painful and should not be attempted.

- Use a silver nitrate stick applied *through* an aural speculum. This protects the skin of the nasal vestibule from inadvertent cautery and subsequent scarring.

- Cauterize around the vessel as well as directly onto the vessel. Simply applying the stick directly onto the vessel can sometimes result in a bleed, making it more difficult to cauterize the area effectively and increasing the risk of the chemical spreading onto the skin of the upper lip.

Nasal packing

This is most likely to be used for a posterior bleed in an older patient where first-aid measures have failed. Packing the nose with ribbon gauze has been a traditional method used in ENT departments. However, a Merocel nasal pack is a quick and easy alternative in all but the most severe bleeds.

The principle of the Merocel pack is similar to that of the otowick: it is hard and rigid and can be slid into the nose relatively easily. When saline is dripped onto it the pack expands and becomes soft, filling the nasal cavity and producing a degree of tamponade which will control the bleeding. A Merocel pack is supplied with a string attached to the anterior end. This can be fixed to the patient's cheek to ensure the pack does not dislodge into the nasopharynx and obstruct the airway.

The throat

Removing a foreign body

Sharp objects such as fish bones can stick anywhere, but they are most commonly found in the tonsil and tongue base. It is therefore worth at least looking at the back of the mouth if the patient gives a history of fish bone ingestion.

If the bone is seen in this area, it is quite feasible to remove it with a suitable instrument, adequate light source and a co-operative patient. It is often worth asking the patient to protrude and then hold his or her own tongue (the family practitioner then has both hands free).

Chapter 7

Shared care in practice: case studies

Case 1:   Discharging, itchy ear

Case 2:   Discharging ear, hearing loss

Case 3:   Deafness in children

Case 4:   Nasal obstruction in children

Case 5:   Nasal obstruction in adults

Case 6:   Epistaxis

Case 7:   Dysphagia

Case 8:   Lateral neck lump

Case 9:   Neck lump below the ear lobe

Case 10:   Danger signs in ENT

Case I: Discharging, 'itchy' ear

A 28-year-old woman returned from a holiday in the Caribbean with a 2-week history of irritation and discharge from the right ear. There was no previous history of ear problems. On examination the ear canal was oedematous and full of debris, not allowing a view of the tympanic membrane. Tuning fork tests of hearing (positive Rinne test on the right, Weber lateralized to the right) suggested a mild conductive hearing loss on the right. How would you proceed?

Family practitioner. The history of discharge in combination with irritation is very suggestive of an otitis externa. However, as there is no view of the eardrum it is impossible to exclude the possibility that the discharge is related to an underlying chronic suppurative otitis media (CSOM) and that this patient has developed a secondary otitis externa.

First-line management of the discharging ear (whatever the underlying cause) involves removing debris and treatment with topical antibiotic/steroid ear drops, together with advice about keeping the ears dry. In many cases of otitis externa this regime will lead to resolution of the problem, although the condition may recur from time to time.

If the discharge was secondary to an underlying perforation (CSOM) then the topical treatment will often produce a dry ear. On review a good view of the tympanic membrane will be obtained and the presence of the perforation can be confirmed.

Otolaryngologist. Otitis externa is often referred to as 'tropical ear', 'swimmer's ear' or 'surfer's ear'. The history is highly suggestive of an otitis externa and the majority of straightforward cases can be managed in family practice. If the ear canal is so swollen that the drops are unlikely to penetrate, then the use of an otowick for a few days will help.

Otitis externa is the commonest reason for patients to visit the

ENT department. If the condition continues to cause troublesome symptoms despite a thorough trial of first-line management, then referral is appropriate.

In the ENT department the ear can be cleaned very effectively using a microscope and suction, and often this aural toilet is the most important part of management. Cleaning usually allows inspection of the tympanic membrane and rules out the presence of a perforation. A pure tone audiogram (if performed) will show only a mild 20–30 dB conductive hearing loss.

As in family practice, initial medical treatment will involve antibiotic/steroid ear drops and advice about keeping the ear dry. If the ear canal is very swollen then an otowick may be required to allow the ear drops to penetrate.

After multiple antibiotic/steroid ear drops, some patients develop a secondary fungal otitis externa. This may be suspected on inspection under the microscope (fungal spores can often be seen). In such a case it may be reasonable to take a swab for culture to confirm the diagnosis and start an antifungal ear drop such as clotrimazole.

Occasionally the otitis externa is so severe (or has spread to produce a secondary perichondritis of the pinna) that the patient requires admission for parenteral antibiotics as well as local treatment.

In rare cases, diabetic and immunocompromised patients develop an aggressive otitis externa with intense pain and the possibility of multiple cranial neuropathies as a result of a spreading skull base 'osteomyelitis'. This is a life-threatening condition which requires hospital admission and aggressive medical treatment.

Case 2: Discharging ear, hearing loss

A 38-year-old mechanic presents with a 3-week history of painless discharge from his left ear. He has noticed problems with his hearing in this ear over the past 3 years and now cannot use the telephone on this side. He had a history of glue ear as a child and has had five episodes of discharge from the ear in the past 4 years.

On examination it was impossible to obtain an adequate view of the eardrum because of the presence of the discharge. Tuning fork tests of hearing (negative Rinne test on the left, Weber lateralized to the left) suggested a significant conductive hearing loss in the left ear. The fistula test was negative and the facial nerve intact. How would you manage this patient?

Family practitioner. It can be difficult to know whether the discharge is secondary to a problem of the ear canal (otitis externa) or the middle ear (CSOM). However, topical treatment with antibiotic/steroid ear drops may help whatever the underlying pathology.

In this case the history of glue ear as a child and the previous history of recurrent painless otorrhoea suggests it is more likely to be related to CSOM. Indeed, the significant hearing loss is also more likely to be related to middle ear pathology than to an otitis externa (which usually produces a mild hearing loss).

The ear drops may allow a better examination of the tympanic membrane on review 2 weeks later. If the ear is dry and a central perforation is noted (i.e. a margin of eardrum can clearly be seen around the perforation) then no referral may be required (unless the patient wishes to consider surgical repair or a hearing aid). If the ear is still wet and no clear view of the eardrum is obtained, or if a marginal perforation (no rim of eardrum visible or the perforation is posterior or in the attic) is noted then ENT referral is indicated.

Otolaryngologist. The history of recurrent painless discharge (with no associated irritation) is suggestive of CSOM. In the ENT department, with the benefit of the microscope and ear suction, it should be possible to visualize the eardrum and establish the diagnosis.

In the case of a central perforation a pure tone audiogram will show a conductive hearing loss of approximately 30–50 dB. Surgery is not essential but may be an option. Myringoplasty (repair of the eardrum) is not always 100% successful, but if it does close the hole then it would eliminate the bouts of discharge. It may or may not lead to an improvement in the hearing.

In the case of a marginal perforation (usually associated with a cholesteatoma) a pure tone audiogram may show a greater conductive hearing loss. Cholesteatoma is capable of destroying the ossicular chain and then a conductive loss of greater than 60 dB may be seen. Surgery in the form of a mastoid operation would be indicated to avoid the potential complications of the condition (e.g. facial palsy, meningitis, brain abscess).

Case 3: Deafness in children

A 4-year-old girl was brought to the surgery by her mother with a 2-month history of possible hearing loss noted by both her parents and her nursery teacher. There was no family history of deafness.

On examination she had bilateral glue ear and tympanometry performed in the surgery showed flat traces bilaterally. What advice would you give to her parents?

Family practitioner. Glue ear is the commonest cause of a hearing loss in children. It is seasonal, being more common during the winter and tending to resolve in the summer (except in atopic individuals). It is also age-related, being more common in younger children (i.e. children do outgrow the problem). In approximately 60% of children, glue ear will resolve spontaneously over a 3-month period.

In view of the above, there is a very good case for a period of watchful waiting, reviewing the situation over 3 months (use of an Otovent balloon to encourage Eustachian tube function over that time may be worthwhile). If there is no improvement after that time then referral is indicated. Referral at an earlier stage may be appropriate if there are other problems such as associated severe otalgia, very frequent acute otitis media, significant speech delay (in younger children) or educational problems (in older children).

Otolaryngologist. A flat tympanogram may indicate the presence of middle ear fluid (as well as wax in the ear canal or perforation of the eardrum) but it gives no indication of hearing thresholds. In view of this, if a child is referred with probable glue ear the hearing will be assessed to help confirm the diagnosis. Usually glue ear produces a 30–40 dB conductive hearing loss. If the loss is greater than this, then one must consider the possibility that there may be an underlying sensorineural hearing loss as well as the glue ear. In this situation it may be still appropriate to treat the glue ear but the possibility of further treatment (e.g. a hearing aid) needs to be considered.

There are no randomized controlled trials to show that any medical treatment accelerates the natural resolution rate of this condition. The management options therefore include watchful waiting, surgical treatment or a hearing aid.

In view of the 60% natural resolution rate, watchful waiting is a reasonable option. However, many children referred to the ENT department have already been through this exercise with their own family practitioners.

Surgical treatment involves bilateral grommet insertion (in some cases combined with adenoidectomy): this is the commonest operation performed in children in this country. When indicated it is usually highly effective in bringing the hearing back to normal levels. The grommets remain in place for about 12 months and approximately 75% of children will require no further grommets (i.e. by the time the grommets have been extruded the child will have outgrown the problem).

A hearing aid does not involve hospital admission or anaesthesia. It will bring the hearing levels up and can be used until the condition resolves.

The choice of management option depends on individual circumstances together with the wishes of the parents. There may be greater pressure for the surgical option if the hearing loss is producing speech delay, or educational or behavioural problems.

Case 4: Nasal obstruction in children

A 6-year-old boy was brought to the surgery by his parents with a history of intermittent nasal obstruction and continual sniffing. He snored at night but there was nothing in the history to suggest obstructive sleep apnoea. His parents wished to know whether removal of his adenoids would help the situation. How would you answer this question?

Family practitioner. This boy's nasal obstruction could be related to large adenoids (although in that case the nasal obstruction would be more likely to be persistent rather than intermittent) but may also be related to other problems such as rhinitis. It might therefore be worthwhile trying a therapeutic trial of topical nasal steroids (e.g. Flixonase).

The adenoids tend to shrink in size from the age of 7–9 years onwards, and may well have disappeared by the late teens/early twenties. In view of this, adenoidectomy is not essential (under any circumstances). Although it is possible it may help his nasal airway to some extent, it is difficult to know if it would do anything as far as his sniffing is concerned.

In view of the above I would advise avoiding surgery if possible.

Otolaryngologist. Assessment of the nasal airway and examination of the nose and postnasal space may throw some light on the underlying cause of the nasal obstruction. In a co-operative child, the adenoids may be visualized using a postnasal space mirror, and their size (together with the adequacy of the nasopharyngeal airway) may be assessed on a lateral postnasal space radiograph.

If the adenoids are large then it would be possible to advise the parents that adenoidectomy might help the nasal airway. It is less likely to be helpful as far as his sniffing is concerned. However, the parents should also be informed that his current symptoms will not harm their son, and that as he gets older his adenoids will shrink in size (and thus his airway should improve). It should be pointed out to them that adenoidectomy is not an essential procedure, and that surgery carries with it risks of morbidity — the commonest complication of this procedure is bleeding (incidence 1–2%).

If the adenoids are large and the parents feel strongly that they wish their son to undergo surgery, I would place his name on the list for adenoidectomy. However, for simple nasal obstruction with no other symptoms I would recommend avoiding surgery wherever possible.

Case 5: Nasal obstruction in adults

A 42-year-old man complained of increasing bilateral nasal obstruction which had come on over the past 2 years. More recently he had noticed problems with his senses of smell and taste. Examination in the surgery confirmed bilateral nasal obstruction and the presence of bilateral nasal polyps (mobile when touched with a probe and non-tender). How do you manage this problem?

Family practitioner. Because bilateral nasal polyps have been identified it is possible to be confident that the problem is not neoplastic.

Treatment in family practice will be with oral and/or topical nasal steroids. If symptoms are severe then a short course of oral steroids (if not contraindicated) followed by long-term topical nasal steroids may be appropriate. If they are less severe, then topical nasal steroids alone may be sufficient.

The choice of topical nasal steroid lies between betamethasone nose drops or one of the nasal steroid sprays – often the drops are more effective, although less convenient to use. Long term use of betamethasone nose drops is associated with some systemic absorption, and in rare cases has been associated with Cushingoid effects over a period of years. A spray, therefore, may be a more appropriate long-term treatment. Indeed, if topical steroids are effective they will need to be used on a regular basis or the polyps will recur.

If medical treatment fails to control the symptoms then referral will be necessary.

Otolaryngologist. The pathogenesis of simple nasal polyps is not understood. Whatever treatment modality is used they will recur at some point (the period before which they recur is very variable and varies from months to decades), but there is evidence that using topical nasal steroids will provide a longer polyp-free interval.

Surgery for simple nasal polyps is indicated only if the patient feels their symptoms warrant it. It is not essential, and in many long-term cases is only used when the patient can no longer manage. In the past, surgery has involved simple removal of polyps via the nose; more recently rigid nasal endoscopes have allowed better visualization peroperatively.

Case 6: Epistaxis

A 72-year-old man presents with active bleeding from the right side of his nose that started 3 hours earlier. It has not stopped despite his pinching his nostrils tightly and using a bag of frozen peas applied to the nasal bridge. How should this problem be managed?

Family practitioner. It may be worth trying to identify a bleeding point and cauterising the nose after applying a local anaesthetic. However, in order to do this a good light source, suction and probably some experience obtained within an ENT department at some point during training are needed. If these are not available, it may be more sensible to opt to place an anterior nasal pack in an attempt to control the bleeding, and then possibly refer the patient onto the ENT department. A Merocel nasal pack is probably the easiest and most effective way of achieving this.

Although some family practitioner units would place an anterior nasal pack and allow the patient to go home (removing the pack in the surgery the following day), it may be preferable to refer any patient with an anterior pack to the ENT department for consideration for hospital admission.

Otolaryngologist. Epistaxis is the commonest reason for emergency admission to an ENT ward. A severe epistaxis is a life-threatening situation and obviously the patient is resuscitated if in shock.

If the patient arrives with an anterior Merocel pack that has controlled the bleed then he would probably simply be admitted and put on bed rest, the pack being removed the following day. On admission, blood would be taken to check clotting studies and haemoglobin (and to group and save if felt necessary).

If the anterior pack was not controlling the bleed then other options are available. The bleeding point might be identified with the aid of a nasal endoscope and electrocautery used to arrest the bleed. The nose could be packed with a posterior pack (often a Foley catheter is used with the balloon blown up within the nasopharynx to tamponade the posterior part of the nose) as well as an anterior nasal pack. If an anterior and posterior pack failed to control the bleed, the nose would be packed under general anaesthetic (again using anterior and posterior packs). If packing under anaesthetic failed to control the bleed, clipping of vessels (external carotid artery, maxillary artery, ethmoidal arteries) would be used together with packing.

Case 7: Dysphagia

A 39-year-old woman presents with a 6-week history of a feeling of a lump in her throat. The feeling is not present at all times and she localizes it to the level of the suprasternal notch. She has no associated hoarseness or true dysphagia, and no symptoms to suggest oesophageal reflux. Examination of the oral cavity, oropharynx and neck are normal. How would you manage this patient?

Family practitioner. The symptoms are characteristic of globus pharyngeus. As her symptoms have been present for 6 weeks it may be reasonable to arrange a barium swallow to assess the hypopharynx and upper oesophagus. If this proves normal, then it may be that this will be enough reassurance to help her. However, if the symptoms persist despite the normal barium swallow, then referral will be necessary to allow visualization of the larynx and hypopharynx. However unlikely, more serious pathology can sometimes present with globus type symptoms.

Otolaryngologist. The symptoms are indeed characteristic of globus pharyngeus (the underlying pathology in this condition is not understood). If the patient were referred with a normal barium swallow then the larynx and hypopharynx would be assessed by indirect laryngoscopy or with a flexible nasolaryngoscope. Rarely tongue base and laryngopharyngeal tumours can present with globus symptoms alone.

Although the larynx can be assessed adequately using these techniques, it is very difficult to assess the hypopharynx fully except by using a rigid endoscope under general anaesthesia. If the patient's symptoms persist, it is therefore sometimes justified to perform this procedure.

Case 8: Lateral neck lump

A 52-year-old smoker presents with a 2-month history of a painless lump in the lateral aspect of the left neck. On direct questioning he admits to a mild foreign body sensation in his throat and some soreness. On examination the only abnormal finding is a firm 3 x 4 cm left mid-cervical lymph node. What are the next steps?

Family practitioner. Any firm painless lateral neck lump appearing in an adult is metastatic cancer until proved otherwise. Urgent referral is indicated.

Otolaryngologist. Many surgical specialities see patients with lumps in the neck. However, if the lump is metastatic squamous cell carcinoma within a lymph node, then the primary is usually within the upper aero-digestive tract. ENT surgeons are trained to examine this area and are well qualified to assess whether there is an associated primary within the head and neck.

In this case this man would be seen urgently and given a full ENT assessment. If the lump were thought to be a malignant node, then particular attention would be paid to the nasopharynx, tongue base, tonsil and hypopharynx, which are all potential primary sites.

In view of this man's symptoms it is most likely that he has a primary carcinoma of the tongue base/tonsil/hypopharynx with a metastatic cervical lymph node.

A fine-needle aspiration cytology (FNAC) would be performed on the lump. If it was found to contain squamous carcinoma cells, the patient would be admitted for an endoscopy under general anaesthetic of the whole of the upper aero-digestive tract (panendoscopy) in an attempt to identify the primary. If no obvious primary were seen then biopsies would still be taken from the left nasopharynx, left tongue base, left tonsil (possibly the left tonsil would be removed totally for histological examination) and left hypopharynx to exclude the possibility of any of these being the primary site.

Management of any identified primary site and associated lymph node would involve a combination of surgery and radiotherapy.

Case 9: Neck lump below the ear lobe

A 27-year-old woman presents with a small 1–2 cm diameter lump at the angle of the jaw on the right side, situated just below the ear lobe. She thinks it may have been present for about 12 months and that it has not increased in size over that time. It is not painful and does not vary in size when eating. Her facial nerve function is normal and the rest of her ENT examination is unremarkable. How do you manage this problem?

Family practitioner. The history is more suggestive of a neoplastic rather than an inflammatory pathology. Essentially a lump in this position could be arising from:

- skin and subcutaneous tissues (e.g. lipoma/sebaceous cyst)
- congenital remnants (branchial cyst/arch abnormalities)
- salivary gland (this is the characteristic position for parotid pathology)
- blood vessels (carotid body tumour)
- nerves (benign tumours such as neuromas)
- lymph nodes (primary neoplasm/lymphoma or secondary neoplasm).

If it was possible to be convinced that it was arising within skin then it might be reasonable to excise it under local anaesthetic in the surgery. In view of the length of the history, all of the other possible pathologies require referral for a full head and neck examination and further investigation.

Otolaryngologist. In view of the length of history and the position of the lump it is most likely that this will prove to be a benign tumour within the parotid gland. All of the other pathologies mentioned above are possible but are less common in this position. If the tumour is positioned in the superficial part of the parotid gland then on palpation it can feel extremely superficial, and it is possible to become convinced that it is arising within the skin and subcutaneous tissue. However, any lump around the ear lobe is within the parotid until proved otherwise. Attempting to remove a sebaceous cyst under local anaesthetic that turns out to be a tumour within the parotid can result in a complete facial palsy.

If the rest of the ENT examination is normal, then fine-needle aspiration cytology (FNAC) will be performed. FNAC is approximately 80% accurate and will often confirm a benign tumour of salivary gland origin, but may also indicate a malignant tumour of salivary gland origin or lymphoma. It may be therapeutic in the case of a parotid cyst. An MRI scan will be arranged to confirm that the lump is within the parotid.

The patient can be reviewed when the results of the investigations are available, and her further management discussed. If all investigations suggest it is a benign parotid tumour, then surgery is indicated in a woman of this age.

Surgery would be recommended for several reasons. Although FNAC is helpful, it cannot rule out malignancy completely. Even if this patient's tumour is benign, there are recorded cases of malignant change within a benign tumour. In addition, the larger the tumour then the greater the risk to the facial nerve. In a young patient one can anticipate a slow increase in tumour size, so it is highly likely that she will require surgery at some stage in her life. Delaying surgery until the tumour is larger means that the risk of damage to the facial nerve will be greater.

The patient would be counselled about the risks of surgery, the most important of which includes damage to the facial nerve.

In older patients where there are contraindications to surgery, it may be reasonable to simply monitor the lump and only consider operating if there are pressing reasons, e.g. if there is a rapid increase in size raising the possibility of a malignant rather than a benign neoplastic process.

Case 10: Danger signs in ENT

The 51-year-old manager of the local Chinese restaurant (who is Hong Kong Chinese) presents with a history of a gradually progressive right-sided hearing loss. There is nothing in the history to suggest it was preceded by an upper respiratory tract infection. On examination it is thought that he may have a right middle ear effusion, and tuning fork tests suggest a mild conductive hearing loss on the right. Would it be reasonable to reassure him that it will probably resolve and review him in a few weeks time?

Family practitioner. Many middle ear effusions are secondary to upper respiratory tract infections and under these circumstances (especially when bilateral) it would be very reasonable to review the situation in a few weeks, as the majority will resolve spontaneously. However, in this case the fact that he is Chinese is highly relevant — nasopharyngeal carcinoma is the commonest form of cancer in the Southern Chinese. This may present in several ways, but a unilateral middle ear effusion secondary to obstruction of the Eustachian tube is one presentation. This man requires urgent referral to the ENT department.

Otolaryngologist. As mentioned above, nasopharyngeal carcinoma (NPC) is the commonest form of malignancy in the Southern Chinese. Indeed in Hong Kong all patients attending the ENT department have NPC until proved otherwise.

The presentation of this condition may involve one or more of the following:
- ear – unilateral middle ear effusion
- nose – obstruction, epistaxis
- neck – secondary lymphadenopathy
- cranial neuropathies – III, IV, V, VI as well as X and XII.

When referred to the ENT department this patient would undergo a full head and neck examination as well as audiology and, in particular, his nasopharynx would be assessed with a flexible or rigid endoscope.

It is most likely that a mucosal lesion would be seen in the region of the Eustachian tube cushion and he would be admitted for an examination under anaesthesia and biopsy of the nasopharynx to obtain histological confirmation of the diagnosis. Some surgeons would drain the middle ear fluid under the same anaesthetic, and insert a grommet into the right ear in an attempt to improve his hearing.

If the tumour is not too extensive and there is no associated lymphadenopathy then first-line management would involve a course of radical radiotherapy.

Index

A

acoustic neuroma 54, 67, 72, 76
  MRI scan 51
adenoidal hypertrophy 18
adenoidectomy, indications 122
adenotonsillectomy 127
ageusia 110
air conduction (AC) 6
airway, continuous positive
  airway pressure
  (CPAP) 126
allergic rhinitis 95–6
  seasonal allergens 96
allergy tests 19
alpha-adrenoceptor agonists 99
anti-streptolysin O (ASO) titre
  118
  sore throat 118
antibiotics, acute sore throat
  118–19
anticholinergics, topical 100
antihistamines 99–100
aphthous stomatitis 109
  recurrent 111–12
apnoea, obstructive sleep
  124–8
ASOM see otitis media, acute
  suppurative
astemizole 99
attico-antral chronic otitis
  media 40–1
audiometry 8–11
  impedance audiometry
    10–11
  pure tone audiograms 10,
    50, 69
  tympanometry 10–11
audiovestibular symptoms 51
aural polyps 25
auricular haematoma 22–3,
  149–50, 152
auriscope, fibreoptic 2

B

barium swallow 14
barotrauma, acute 28–9, 151–2
basal cell carcinoma, pinna 23
bat ears 21
beclomethasone dipropionate
  93, 98

Bell's palsy (idiopathic facial
  paralysis) 80, 82
  assessment and management
    82–3
  specialist referral 83–4
benign paroxysmal positional
  vertigo (BPPV) 67
  positional testing 69
  referral 74
  symptoms 70
blast injuries, inner/middle ear
  151
blood test, monospot 14
bone conduction (BC) 6
BPPV (benign paroxysmal
  positional vertigo),
  positional testing 69
branchial cyst 146, 147

C

C-reactive protein (CRP) 118
caloric tests 69
candidiasis, oral 113
case studies 173–80
  childhood nasal obstruction
    179–80
  deafness in childhood 177–9
  discharging ear, hearing loss
    175–7
  dysphagia 183–4
  ear lobe 185–7
  ENT referral, danger signs
    187–8
  epistaxis 181–3
  itchy ear, discharging 174–5
cauliflower ear 22–3
cerebral/cerebellar abscess 39
cetirizine 99
cholesteatoma 33, 44, 67
  chronic otitis media 40, 55
chorda tympani 79
chronic suppurative otitis media
  see otitis media (CSOM)
ciliary function tests 19
cochlear implants 62–3
  constituents 63
conductive deafness 46, 49,
  55–6, 58
continuous positive airway
  pressure (CPAP) 126
corticosteroids, allergic rhinitis
  98

Coxsackie virus infection
  112
croup (laryngotracheo-
  bronchitis) 138–9
CSOM see otitis media, chronic
  suppurative
CT scans
  chronic rhinosinusitis 104
  neck, assessment
    tumour/abscess
    position 14
  paranasal sinuses 18
cystic hygroma 146

D

danger signs
  ENT emergencies 161–3
  ENT referral, case study
    187–8
  nasal emergencies 162
  oropharyngeal emergency
    163
deafness see hearing loss
dental disease, local 104
dental pain 104–5
dermal cyst 145
dexamethasone, nasal polyps
  93
diabetes, necrotizing
  (malignant) otitis
  externa 36
diphtheria 117
distraction test 4–5
dizziness
  associated symptoms 67
  duration 67
  examination and assessment
    69–70
  general practice examination,
    examples 67–9
  historical significance 66–7
  non-otological/otological
    causes 65
  specialist referral 74
  see also vertigo
dysphagia 134
  acute 130
  assessment and diagnosis
    128–9
  case study 183–4
  causes 130
  chronic 130

ENT department assessment
130
examination and referral
129–30
foreign body-associated,
investigations 129
intrinsic lesions 131–2
specialist referral 133
dysphonia, organic causes
classified 134

E

ear, danger signs and
symptoms 162
ear canal 2, 21–3, 33, 52
carcinoma 29
congenital abnormalities
23–4
external meatus injury 150–1
osteoma 25
ear discharge 32–43
chronic suppurative otitis
media (CSOM) 33
dry-mopping discharge 168
examination and diagnosis
32–3
hearing loss, case study
175–7
itchy ear, case study 174–5
sources of discharge and
diagnoses 32
ear examination 1–3
danger signs and symptoms
161–2
deafness in childhood, case
study 177–9
dry-mopping discharge 168
ear infection, specialist
referral 23
ear wick insertion 36–7, 168
external ear 21–3
bat ears 21
cauliflower ear 22–3
referral 26
'swimmer's ear' 34
'tropical ear' 34
foreign body removal
examination 24, 150
instruments 168–9
syringing 168
hearing loss, discharging
ear, case study 175–7
inner/middle ear injury 73,
151–2
blast injuries 151
head injury 152
otitic barotrauma 151–2
microtia 21
polyps 2, 25

referral considerations 26, 169
specialist referral 57
syringing 150, 167–8
contraindications 25, 150
see also hearing loss; otalgia;
otitis media
ear lobe, case study 185–7
ear protection 53
ear rupture
oval window 73
round window, specialist
referral 73
ear surgery, scar positions 1
ear syringing 167–8
contraindications 25, 150
indications 33, 150
ear trauma 24, 149–52
eardrum perforation 41, 52
specialist referral 153
ear tumours/neoplasia 23, 25,
29
ear wax 24–5, 167
ear wick insertion 36–7, 168
earache
grommet 39
see also otalgia
emergencies see danger signs
endolymphatic hydrops
(Menière's disease) 50,
67, 71–2
specialist referral 72
symptoms 71–2
endoscope, rigid nasal 13,
16–17, 100
endotracheal intubation 142
ENT emergencies, danger signs
and symptoms 161–3,
187–8
ENT referral, danger signs, case
study 187–8
ephedrine 99
epiglottitis 141
acute 140
epistaxis 85–8
anterior bleed 86–7
management 88
case study 181–3
ENT department
management 88
general causes 86
local causes, Little's area
85–6
management 86
persisting active bleeding 87
posterior bleeding 87
management 88
recurrent 88
specialist referral 89
Eustachian tube dysfunction,
chronic 41
extratemporal nerve 79

F

facial nerve anatomy 78–9
facial nerve paralysis 39, 78–84,
81
assessment 79–84
flow chart 81
Bell's palsy (idiopathic facial
paralysis) 80–4
lower motor neurone (LMN)
lesion, causes 82
management 83
referral 83–4, 152
facial pain 102–7
atypical 106
causes classified 103–6
dental pain 104–5
sites causing referred pain 102
specialist referral 107
family practice procedures
ear
dry-mopping discharge 168
foreign body removal
instruments 168–9
syringing 168
paediatric referral 169
syringing 167–8
hearing loss
clinical tests 4–9
older children and adults
5–9
nasal packing 170
nose
foreign body removal 169
nasal cautery 169–70
throat, foreign body removal
171
see also foreign bodies
FESS (functional endoscopic
sinus surgery) 104
fibreoptic auriscope 2
Foley urethral catheter 88
foreign bodies
dysphagia 129
ear canal 150
ear examination 24
instruments 168–9
inhaled, oropharyngeal
trauma 158
nasal 169
nasal fractures 155–6
oropharyngeal, removal 171
radiography 158
stridor 141
swallowed, oropharyngeal
trauma 158–9
functional endoscopic sinus
surgery (FESS) 104
fungal infections, oral
ulceration 112
furunculosis 28

G

glomerulonephritis, acute 120
glossitis, median rhomboid
114
glossopharyngeal neuralgia 106
glue ear *see* otitis media
GP practice procedures *see*
family practice
procedures
grommets 48
earache relief 39
infected 42, 44

H

haematoma
auricular 22–3, 149–50, 152
nasal septum 154
halitosis 110
Hallpike test 68
hard palate, squamous cell
carcinoma 112
hay fever *see* allergic rhinitis
head injuries 152
head and neck cancer 164–6
presenting features 165–6
see also neck lumps
headaches
cluster 105
migraine 105
tension 106
hearing aids 48, 57–62
audiology department
referral 61
electronic air conduction
components 59
private dispensers 61
problems associated 58–9
sources 61–3
specialist referral 61, 64
types 60
behind the ear (BE) 60
body worn aids 60
bone conduction aids 60
'in the ear' 60
hearing examination 3–11
hearing loss
adults 5–9, 49–56
audiometry 8–11
impedance audiometry
10–11
pure tone audiograms
9–10
bilateral >35dB, referral 57,
64
childhood 44–8
case study 177–9
referral 49
risk factors 45

clinical tests 4–9
cochlear implants 62–3
conductive deafness 46, 49,
55–6, 58
pathology 3, 4
referral 57, 64
cooperative/performance
tests 5
diagnoses and history 50–1
discharging ear, case study
175–7
distraction test 4–5
environmental aids 62
free field speech test 5
handicap associated 4
lip-reading 62
older children and adults 5–9
performance test 5
referral consideration 57, 61,
64
Rinne test 6–8
sensorineural deafness 3, 49,
53–5
referral 57
severity of loss 3
sign language 62
specialist referral 64
sudden (idiopathic)
sensorineural 54–5
tuning fork tests 6–8
type, Rinne/Weber
combination 8
type and severity 3
Weber tests 7–8
whisper test 50
young children 4
Heimlich manoeuvre 141
herpes stomatitis 112
herpes zoster oticus 29
HIV infection and AIDS 112, 118
hoarseness 133–7
assessment and diagnosis
133–4
benign neoplasia 135–6
chronic laryngitis 135
ENT department examination
134–5
malignant neoplasia 136
specialist referral 138
vocal cord examination 134
Hopkins' optical rod system
nasendoscope 16–17,
100
hormone replacement therapy
(HRT) 126
human papillomavirus 135

I

IgE, radioallergosorbent test
(RAST) 19

immunocompromised patient,
necrotizing (malignant)
otitis externa 36
impedance audiometry 10–11
infectious mononucleosis 117
intracranial nerve 79
intratemporal nerve 79

J

Jobson Horne probe 33

L

labyrinthine failure
acute 67
symptoms and treatment
71
labyrinthitis 39, 54
acute, specialist referral 74
laryngeal examination 12–13
indirect laryngoscopy 12
laryngeal neoplasia 135–6
laryngeal papillomata 141
laryngeal trauma 141
laryngeal web 140
laryngitis, chronic 135
laryngomalacia 140
laryngoscopy
direct laryngoscopy 135
fibreoptic laryngoscopy 135
indirect laryngoscopy 135
laryngotomy 142
laryngotracheobronchitis
(croup) 138–9
lateral sinus thrombosis 39
leucoplakia of tongue 113
lichen planus 113
lip-reading 52, 62
Little's area, nasal septum,
epistaxis local causes
85–6
lower motor neurone (LMN)
lesions 79–80, 82

M

mastoid cavity, infected 42
mastoiditis 33, 39, 42
median rhomboid glossitis 114
Menière's disease
(endolymphatic
hydrops) 50, 67, 71–2
referral 72
specialist referral 72, 74
meningitis 39
Merocel nasal pack 87, 170
microtia 21, 23
middle ear, perforations 52

migraine 105
mononucleosis 117
mouth cancer 112–13
MRI scans 69
    acoustic neuroma exclusion
        51, 55
    nasal tumours 18
    neck, assessment tumour/
        abscess position 14
myringitis bullosa 28
myringoplasty 55

N

nasal angiofibroma 86
nasal cautery 87, 169–70
nasal cycle, normal 90
nasal deformity 154
nasal emergencies 153–6
    danger signs and symptoms
        162
nasal examination 15–17
    airflow assessment 16
    ENT department 18, 91
    epistaxis 85–8
    nasal cavity 16–17
nasal fractures 83, 153–4
    foreign bodies 155–6
    treatment 154–5
nasal neoplasms 86, 94
nasal obstruction 89–94
    assessment 91
    childhood, case study
        179–80
    ENT department assessment
        91
    foreign body removal 169
    history 90
    nasal cautery 169–70
    nose drops, administration
        93
    with runny nose 95–101
        allergen avoidance 97–8
        antihistamines 99–100
        diagnosis and treatment
            96–7
        flow chart for diagnosis
            97
        specialist referral 102
        topical corticosteroids 98–9
    specialist referral 94
nasal packing 170
    Merocel nasal pack 87, 170
nasal polyps 92–4
    examination and referral 92
    medical treatment 92–3
    surgical treatment 93–4
nasal septum
    deviated 91–2
        treatment 91–2

haematoma 154
    post cautery with silver
        nitrate 87
nasal trauma 86, 153–6
    specialist referral 156
nasal tumours 86, 94
nasolaryngoscope, fibreoptic 13
nasopharynx examination
    12–13
neck lumps 143–7
    adult 146–7
        congenital lumps 147
        lateral lumps 146–7
            case study 184–5
        midline lumps 146
        neoplastic lumps 147
        thyroglossal cyst 145
    assessment 145
    ear lobe, case study 185–7
    examination 13–14
    history 143–4
    investigations 144–5
    paediatric 145–6
    referral 148
necrotizing (malignant) otitis
    externa 36
neuralgias 105–6
    central pain 106
neuromuscular disorders,
    swallowing problems
        130–1
noise trauma 53
nose, danger signs and
    symptoms 162
nose bleed see epistaxis
nose drops administration 93
nystagmus
    peripheral 70
    peripheral/central types
        68–9

O

obstructive sleep apnoea (OSA)
    124
    in children 127
    management 126
    sites/causes of obstruction
        125
oesophageal reflux 122
OME see otitis media with
    effusion
operation scars, past, chronic
    otitis media link 52
ophthalmic pain 106
oral cavity
    ageusia 110
    aphthous stomatitis,
        recurrent 111–12
    burning mouth 110

examination 12
haemorrhage 110
halitosis 110
hard palate, squamous cell
    carcinoma 112
infections causing ulceration
    112
lesions 109–15
    black hairy tongue
        114–15
    red lesions 114
    retention cysts 114
        ranula example 114
    torus palatinus 114
    white lesions 113
mouth cancer 112–13
oral candidiasis 113
oral disease, symptoms
    109–10
specialist referral 115, 123
ulceration
    causes 109, 110
    chronic fungal infection
        112
    infections 112
oropharyngeal emergency,
    danger signs and
    symptoms 163
oropharyngeal investigations,
    ENT department 14
oropharyngeal trauma 156–9
    external 157
    inhaled foreign bodies,
        assessment and
        management 158
    specialist referral 160
    swallowed foreign bodies
        assessment and
        management 158–9
        radiograph 158
OSA (obstructive sleep apnoea)
    122–7
osteoma, ear canal 25
osteomyelitis, skull base 36
otalgia 26–31
    causes 27
    malignant disease 31
    non-otological causes 30–1
    osteoarthritis, cervical spine
        31
    otological causes 27–9
    otological/non-otological
        causes 27
    referral conditions 31
    unilateral 134
otitic barotrauma, acute 28–9,
    151–2
otitis externa 23, 28, 33, 34–6
    assessment and
        management, ENT
        referral 42–4

ear canal 35
ENT department, assessment
    and management 42–3
itching 33
necrotizing (malignant) 36
otowick 36–7, 168
pinna skin changes 35
referral 43
severe 32–3
sign 1
otitis media
active suppurative (ASOM)
    40, 32–3
    recurrent ASOM 39
    referral 44
    symptoms examination
        and treatment 37–9
'adhesive' 48
antibiotics 38–9
attico-antral chronic 41
childhood 27
chronic suppurative (CSOM)
    27, 33, 40, 51
    with cholesteatoma 55
    labyrinthitis 73
    referral 44
    tubotympanic/attico-antral
        comparison 40
    with/without
        cholesteatoma 55
complications 39
with effusion (OME, glue
    ear) 44–8, 56, 58
    assessment and
        management 47–8
    conductive hearing loss
        46
    flat tympanogram 47
    tympanic membrane
        appearance 46
otologic (subjective) tinnitus 75
otorrhoea 32–44, 80
    sources of 32
otosclerosis 3, 55–6, 58
ototoxic drugs 53–4
otowick insertion 36–7, 168
oval window ear rupture 73

P

palatal myoclonus 77
palate, squamous cell
    carcinoma 112
papillomavirus 135
paranasal sinuses 18
    CT scan 18
parasympathetic nerve
    interruption 101
parotid gland tumour 82
parotid region, lumps 13

pars flaccida 3
pars tensa 3
Paul-Bunnell blood test 14, 117
perforated eardrum 41, 52
perichondritis infection 23, 28
perilymph fistula 152
peripheral vestibular function,
    caloric tests 69–70
peritonsillar abscess 119
pharyngitis, chronic 122
pharynx
    carcinoma of the
        hypopharynx 147
    examination 12–13
    globus pharyngeus 131–2
    neoplasia 131
    parotid mass, characteristic
        site 147
    peritonsillar abscess 119
    pharyngeal pouch 131
    barium swallow 131
pinna 1
    basal cell carcinoma 23
    congenital abnormalities
        21–2
    injury to 149–50
    neoplasia 23
    see also ear, external
polyps
    aural 25
    nasal 92–4
post-herpetic neuralgia 106
postnasal space examination 18
preauricular granuloma 22
preauricular sinuses 22
presbyacusis 53, 58
    milder hearing loss,
        specialist referral 64
    specialist referral 78
    tinnitus 75
proton pump inhibitor 122
pure tone audiometry 50

Q

quinsy 119

R

radioallergosorbent test (RAST)
    19
Ramsay Hunt syndrome 29
respiratory tract infection,
    recurrent upper 45
retention cysts, oral cavity 114
rheumatic fever, acute 120
rhinitis 90
    allergic rhinitis 95–6
    classified 95–6

ENT department
    management 100–1
    infective 95
    intrinsic 96
    referral 102
rhinitis medicamentosa 99
rhinological disease, malignant
    104
rhinological pain 103–4
rhinometry 19
    acoustic 19
rhinorrhoea, watery 95, 99–100
rhinoscopy, anterior 16
rhinosinusitis, chronic 104
Rinne test 6–8, 46
Romberg test 68
round window ear rupture,
    specialist referral 73

S

scars 1, 52
sensorineural deafness 3, 49,
    53–5, 57
    acoustic neuroma 54
    noise trauma 53
    ototoxic drugs 54
    presbyacusis 53–5
    referral 57
    sudden (idiopathic) 54–5
septal haematoma 154
sign language 62
sinuses
    functional endoscopic sinus
        surgery (FESS) 104
    normal coronal CT scan 19
    paranasal, CT scan 18
    preauricular sinuses 22
    thrombosis, lateral sinus 39
sinusitis 103–4
sleep apnoea 124–8
    indicators 124
    specialist referral 128
snoring 124–6
    causes 125
    management 126
    sites/causes of obstruction
        125
    specialist referral 128
    surgical referral 126, 128
sodium cromoglycate 100
sore throat
    acute sore throat
        antibiotics 118–19
        causes 116
        self-care by patients 118
        treatment 118–19
    anti-streptolysin O (ASO)
        titre 118
    C-reactive protein (CRP) 118

chronic sore throat 122–3
  chronic pharyngitis 122
  diphtheria 117
  examination 12–13
  infectious mononucleosis 117
  Paul-Bunnell tests 117
  rapid antigen tests 118
  swabs 117–18
  see also oropharyngeal
    region; tonsillitis
squamous cell carcinoma, hard
  palate 112
stapedial nerve 79
stomatitis
  aphthous recurrent 109,
    111–12
  primary herpes 112
streptococcal tonsillitis 116–17
stridor 138–42
  adult 141
  age-specific causes 139
  congenital abnormalities
    140–1
  defined 134
  ENT department
    management 141–2
  foreign bodies 141
  management 141–2
  specialist referral 143
  treatment 139
subglottic haemangioma 140
subglottic stenosis 141
superficial petrosal nerve 79
supraglottitis 141
swallowing, neuromuscular
  disorders 130–1
'swimmer's ear' 34
syphilis, oral ulceration 112

T

temporal arteritis 105
temporal bone fractures 152
temporomandibular joint
  dysfunction 31, 104–5
terfenadine 99
throat see oropharyngeal
  region; sore throat;
  tonsillitis
Thudichum's nasal speculum
  16–17

thyroglossal cysts 13, 145
tinnitus 72, 74–7
  drug therapy,
    cause/exacerbation 75
  ear diseases associated 76
  examination and specialist
    referral 76
  management 76–7
  onset 54
  otologic (subjective) 75
  pulsatile 77
  specialist referral 78
  transmitted (objective) 77
  types 74–7
  unilateral 72–3, 78
tongue
  black hairy 114–15
  geographical 114
  leucoplakia 113
  malignancies, referral 113
  median rhomboid glossitis
    114
tonsillectomy
  indications/contraindications
    120–1
  post 30
  postoperative care 121–2
tonsillitis 30
  acute follicular tonsillitis
    116
  acute streptococcal tonsillitis
    116–17
  chronically infected tonsils
    123
  complications 119
topical anticholinergics 100
torus palatinus 114
tracheostomy 142
trigeminal neuralgia 105
'tropical ear' 34
tuberculosis, oral ulceration 112
tubotympanic disease 40–1
tubotympanic/attico-antral
  comparison CSOM
    40–1
tuning fork tests 6–8, 50, 54, 75
tympanic membrane 33–4
  appearance, otitis media
    with effusion 46
  centrally perforated 41
  examination 2
  marginally perforated 41

normal 2
  perforation 52
tympanometry 10–11
  common trace types 10
tympanosclerosis 52

U

ulceration, oral cavity 112
Unterberger test 68
upper airway obstruction,
  stridor 138–42
upper motor neurone (UMN)
  lesion 79–80
uvulopalatopharyngoplasty
  (UPPP) 126
  before/after appearance
    127

V

vagus nerve 136
Valsalva manoeuvre 34
vascular pain, head/neck 105
vasoconstrictors 99
vertigo 54, 65, 72–4
  benign paroxysmal
    positional (BPPV) 67,
    69–70, 74
  episodic 71
  referral 74
  see also dizziness
vestibular neuronitis, symptoms
  and treatment 71
vestibular system, physiology
  66
vidian neurectomy 101
vocal cords
  carcinoma 137
  nodules 136
  paralysis 136–7
  polyp 136

W

Weber tests 7–8

X

xylometazoline 99